Health Communication and the Medical Humanities

AF819146

Drawing upon actual case studies, this book introduces readers to how everyday interactions in the clinic can foster trust and impact diagnoses and reveals how often-overlooked communication processes fundamentally shape healthcare delivery and outcomes.

The book treats communication not as a box to be checked or a skill to be mastered, but as a force that shapes provider and patient identities, a broker of relationships, and a central and pervasive presence in all systems of care. It explores topics such as end-of-life communication, physician burnout, professional hierarchies within healthcare teams, and AI in healthcare. It also integrates examples that extend beyond a U.S. framework, accounting for how different healthcare and political systems impact patient care. Each chapter is written in plain language and invites readers to think critically about what true patient-centered care looks like today.

This book is tailored to both undergraduate and graduate medical humanities, health communication, medical sociology, and bioethics courses and a broad audience of healthcare professionals—from nursing students to attending physicians, technicians, and support staff.

Online resources include links to readings, outside resources, and video components. They are available online at www.routledge.com/9781041102779.

Shelby Forbes is a Teaching Professor in the Department of Social Medicine within the School of Medicine at the University of North Carolina at Chapel Hill, USA.

Michael K. Seifert is an Associate Professor in the Department of Orthopaedics in the School of Medicine at the University of North Carolina at Chapel Hill, USA.

Health Communication and the Medical Humanities

A Case-Based Learning Approach

Shelby Forbes and Michael K. Seifert

Routledge
Taylor & Francis Group
NEW YORK AND LONDON

Designed cover image: Tippapatt/Getty

First published 2027
by Routledge
605 Third Avenue, New York, NY 10158

and by Routledge
4 Park Square, Milton Park, Abingdon, Oxon, OX14 4RN

Routledge is an imprint of the Taylor & Francis Group, an informa business

© 2027 Shelby Forbes and Michael K. Seifert

The right of Shelby Forbes and Michael K. Seifert to be identified as authors of this work has been asserted in accordance with sections 77 and 78 of the Copyright, Designs and Patents Act 1988.

All rights reserved. No part of this book may be reprinted or reproduced or utilised in any form or by any electronic, mechanical, or other means, now known or hereafter invented, including photocopying and recording, or in any information storage or retrieval system, without permission in writing from the publishers.

For Product Safety Concerns and Information please contact our EU representative GPSR@taylorandfrancis.com. Taylor & Francis Verlag GmbH, Kaufingerstraße 24, 80331 München, Germany.

Trademark notice: Product or corporate names may be trademarks or registered trademarks, and are used only for identification and explanation without intent to infringe.

ISBN: 978-1-041-10286-1 (hbk)
ISBN: 978-1-041-10277-9 (pbk)
ISBN: 978-1-003-65430-8 (ebk)

DOI: 10.4324/9781003654308

Typeset in Times New Roman
by KnowledgeWorks Global Ltd.

by Access the Support Material: www.routledge.com/9781041102779.

Contents

About the Authors

Dr. Shelby Forbes holds a PhD in communication, and much of her research focuses on matters of health communication. From examining large-scale public health campaigns to interactions between patients and providers at the local level, Dr. Forbes's academic interests focus on how communication processes influence health outcomes. Dr. Forbes's published work moreover seeks to integrate the field of communication with disability studies for greater health equity across this particular patient population. She teaches social medicine courses to first- through third-year medical students at the University of North Carolina-Chapel Hill. In many ways, this book's interdisciplinary emphasis is the product of these endeavors.

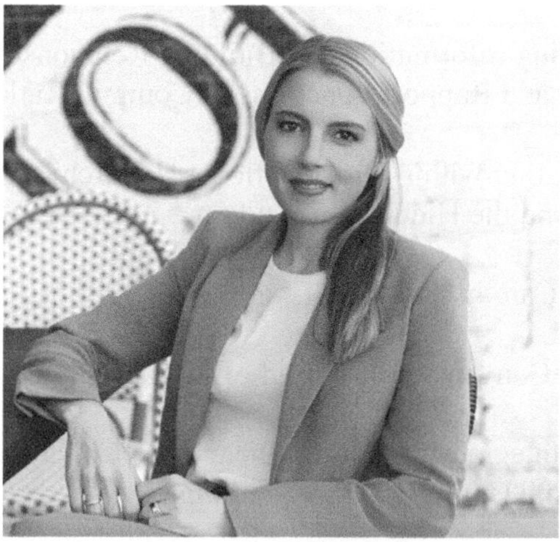

Figure 0.1 A photo of the book's first author, Dr. Shelby Forbes. Photo supplied by the author.

Dr. Michael Seifert holds an MD. He is board certified in Internal Medicine and has a certificate of added qualification in Primary Care Sports Medicine. He brings to this book a wealth of knowledge derived from nine years of clinical practice, first as an internal medicine/primary care physician and then as a sports medicine doctor. As an attending physician and medical educator, he has practiced in two different schools of medicine, as well as trained at three others. He has volunteered on medical mission trips as well as low-cost community care clinics. He has given countless lectures to students, residents, fellows, and the general public using case-based learning (CBL) formats. He has moreover written several articles and book chapters that use individual cases as a framework for teaching, and thus thoroughly recognizes the educational value of this instructional format.

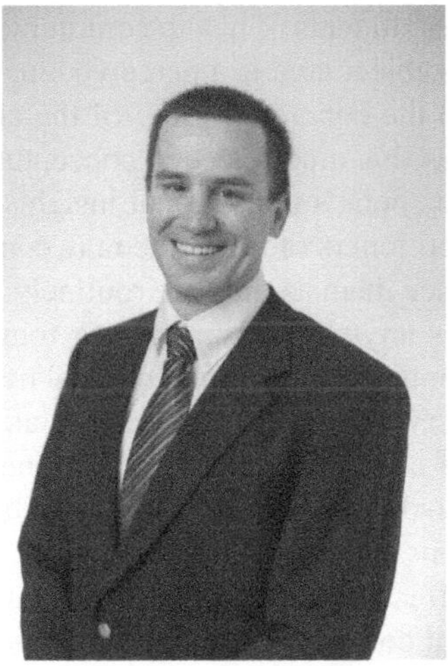

Figure 0.2 A photo of the book's second author, Dr. Michael Seifert. Photo supplied by the author.

Preface

A Note about Case-Based Learning

One of the key difficulties students of health communication and the medical humanities cite about this subject area is a perceived inability to translate abstract theory and constructs to the concrete setting of the clinic. Employing real-life cases, however, serves as this much-needed conceptual bridge. We have therefore chosen to center this book's educational insights around unique examples so that students and practitioners of medicine may come to view these ideas not as mere abstraction but see them as they are routinely manifested in interaction.

Each chapter features anywhere from two to four cases, each of which is informed by actual patients, providers, and clinical events, but with identifying details changed to preserve privacy and confidentiality. We selected the cases that we did because we determined them to be generalizable and representative of communicative challenges and dilemmas that have been exhibited across similar patient populations at multiple points in time.

While these cases differ in their instructional focus, they are united in their common view of clinical communication not as a tool or even a resource, but rather as the very thing that constitutes healthcare itself. Through these cases, readers will come to see communication in clinical practice as unfolding through everyday conversation, patient chart documentation, and institutional routines. Each case serves as a springboard, from which key themes and learning moments are extracted and built upon for further discussion.

The cases featured here also share a similar format. Each includes a description of the patient, their presenting symptoms, chief concern, and a brief social history; their provider(s) and care team, as well as an account of the clinical setting; and a broader description of the healthcare scenario in which these parties find themselves. In this way, they aim to simultaneously showcase the multiple perspectives influencing the delivery of care, and by featuring providers of various roles (e.g., nurses, physician assistants, interns, and attendings), settings (e.g., in-patient and out-patient), and specialties (e.g., oncology, orthopedics, and psychiatry), we invite a diverse audience to engage with the material.

It is important to note, however, that unlike the case-based learning that is often employed to teach students in healthcare professions how to perform differential diagnoses, where there is a clear right or wrong answer, there is decidedly no such thing here. As such, each case is fundamentally interpretative. They are thus not designed to serve as a checklist of best practices but are reflexive exercises that invite the reader to examine the complexity of clinical and organizational life—from how authority is negotiated to how professional identities are constructed, and more. The reader will find that even though actionable recommendations are offered to the prospective clinician, these cases lack a clear-cut resolution, something that reflects an intentional choice on our part. In rejecting a singular "right" answer, we not only attempted to showcase the complexity and nuances of the topics detailed here but emphasize a key tenet of the book: that a one-size-fits-all approach to health communication is destined to fail.

In developing these cases, our goal likewise follows a less-than-linear path. After reflecting on and discussing these cases, we do not expect the reader to become a perfect communicator, simply a more attentive one—one who is prepared to embrace the ambiguities and ethical tensions of healthcare interactions, and to do so in a way that translates to better health outcomes.

1 Rethinking Clinical Care

Case-Based Learning in Health Communication and the Medical Humanities

Case 1

Scenario: It is 11:20 am in an outpatient clinic within the City University School of Medicine (CUSM) healthcare system. Dr. Nelson just finished discussing some concerning lab results with Mrs. Shank, her 10:40 patient. She is joined in clinic by a third-year medical student, James. The medical assistant working with Dr. Nelson, Ann, reminds her that her 11:20 patient, Mr. Liu, has another appointment across town and needs to catch the bus. At 12:00, Dr. Nelson also has a scheduled peer-to-peer phone call with an insurance carrier to have an MRI approved for a patient from last week. She is preparing to step in to see an established patient, Mr. Arnold, her 11:00 appointment. She notes that she has an urgent message on her electronic medical record (EMR), indicating a critical result to review.

Dr. Nelson picks up her open laptop and walks into Mr. Arnold's room. James does the same to see Mr. Liu. Mr. Arnold asks Dr. Nelson if everything is okay because she seems distracted. Mr. Liu expresses disappointment toward James, saying, "I don't want to see the assistant. I have to leave soon, and I was hoping to see the head doctor as soon as possible."

Patients: Mr. Arnold is a 75-year-old male with well-controlled blood pressure and idiopathic peripheral neuropathy who just lost his wife to cancer. He is following up regarding elbow and knee pain that he has been having for several months. Mr. Liu is a 42-year-old male with an unknown medical history. This is his first visit, and he is trying to establish care with Dr. Nelson.

Providers: Dr. Nelson (Figure 1.1) is a general internal medicine provider and assistant professor at CUSM. James, a third-year medical student, is trying to impress Dr. Nelson as he wants a letter of recommendation after the rotation. Ann is the medical assistant working with Dr. Nelson who performs scribing duties for her.

While this case may appear to be written in hyperbole—a caricature of overextended providers—it is a plausible and relatable scenario for many. It is quite

DOI: 10.4324/9781003654308-1

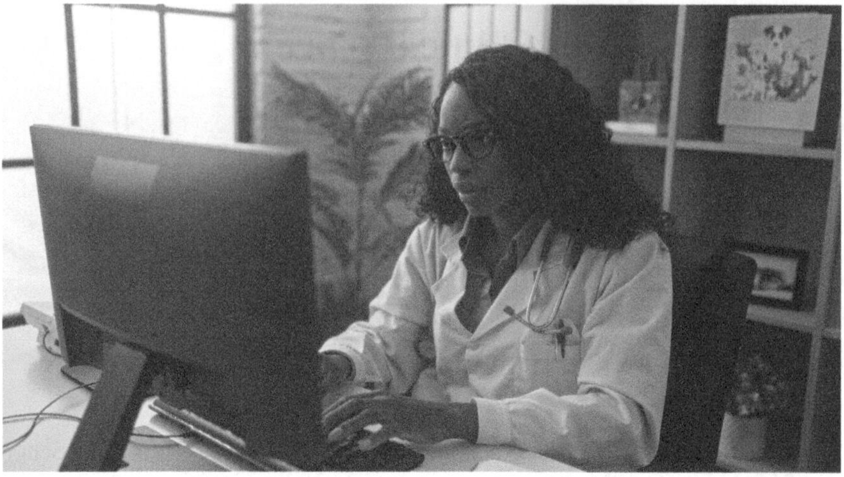

Figure 1.1 A young physician answering patient messages. Photo from Shutterstock.

likely that you, or someone you know, have been a participant in a medical encounter such as this, either as a member of the care team or as a patient on the receiving end of such care. If either Mr. Arnold or Mr. Liu ends up sensing that Dr. Nelson was rushing through their visit, the patient's initial reflex might be to write off Dr. Nelson as a jaded or disinterested provider, or as both distracted and demonstrating subpar "bedside manner." But this case is not meant to be an exercise in doctor-bashing; to engage in such an exercise would not be practically or analytically interesting, nor would it be consistent with the realities of clinical practice. Instead, this case is meant to serve as a window into the multilayered structural constraints that impact the delivery of care.

Within the confines of this single case, we can see the multiple facets of modern healthcare that enter one's practice. The reference to Dr. Nelson being joined by a third-year medical student, for example, illustrates how many providers (particularly those at academic medical institutions) are tasked with not only providing quality healthcare for the patient but also making the encounter an effective learning experience for physicians in training and multiple different members of the care team. Additionally, within this same example, one can observe how **cross-functional communication** across the care team impacts the care provided, as the medical assistant working with Dr. Nelson fulfills the role of a scribe and offers information regarding the next patient's time constraints.

Because of the holistic view it adopts, attending to multiple members of the care team, this book offers insights for medical professionals of all roles and specialities, from first-year medical students, to nursing assistants, to established attendings. Our word choice throughout this text reflects a commitment to making this book relevant to a diverse audience of medical professionals, hence our use of "providers" in lieu of the more specific "physician," "nurse practitioner," and so on. As with this case, and where possible, we try to realistically represent all those individuals involved in patient care, not limiting the episode at hand to the exchanges that occur between doctor and patient.

Returning to the notion of time constraints as they appear in the above case, the unyielding timeline against which clinical interactions often occur is further underscored by the frantic nature of Dr. Nelson's schedule, with patient appointments occurring every 20 minutes or so, at 10:20, 10:40, 11:00, and 11:20. This timetable is a common one, routinely seen in primary care settings, where providers are allocated time slots as brief as 15–20 minutes, in which patients often wish to discuss multiple complex concerns. We can also imagine how difficult it is to adhere to this schedule when providers like Dr. Nelson must review and discuss concerning lab results with the patient. These sorts of discussions often place undue stress on the provider by adding to their **cognitive load**—that is, the mental resources one must employ to complete a particular task (American Psychological Association, 2025).

Then there is the **emotional labor** involved in informing a patient that they have a potentially life-threatening condition. Jeung et al. (2018) define "emotional labor" as emotional work that is "exchanged for something, such as wages." Here, Dr. Nelson is having to do the emotional work of breaking bad news (as indicated by the critical result to review) and consoling what is bound to be a frightened and disheartened patient. Carrying an extensive cognitive load and routinely having to perform emotional labor are two primary factors leading to **provider burnout** (West et al., 2018), a topic that will be addressed in greater depth in Chapter 6 of this book, and a phenomenon that is increasingly becoming a subject of concern within primary care specialties in particular (Rassolian et al., 2017).

Finally, this case emphasizes that communication in the clinic (or hospital, for that matter) happens through various channels, not all of which are face-to-face. The provider must interact with **electronic medical records (EMRs)**, which are a "digital collection of medical information about a person," including their "health history, such as medicines, diagnoses, tests, allergies, immunizations, and treatment plans" (National Cancer Institute, 2025). While EMRs are useful in that they centralize patient health information from disparate sources, they are nonetheless plagued with the more common pitfalls of mediated communication (see Chapter 6), such as a lack of immediate feedback or the inability to clarify content in real time. They are also subject to a distinct lack of contextual features like tone, facial expression, and other **nonverbal communication** indicators,[1] all of which signal how to interpret a message.

This brief excerpt thus touches on several of the themes addressed in this book—from organizational communication to provider burnout, to breaking bad news, to healthcare delivery in the digital age. It exemplifies how a scene that might outwardly be interpreted as a provider unskilled at time management, or one who is indifferent to the depth of patients' various needs, is actually the result of the confluence of multiple institutional and societal structures. This book likewise adopts a more **systemic** view, aiming to view healthcare interactions as the result of multiple systems (i.e., financial, educational, social, and cultural) and communication processes simultaneously at work. Each chapter introduced here is therefore not to be taken in isolation, but should be regarded as intersecting with and building upon the content introduced in all those that came before it, as well as all those after.

In the classroom, the feedback we have received was that while students grasped the importance of learning the theories underpinning certain medical practices and approaches to healthcare delivery, they struggled to see how these theories would show up, in tangible terms, within their clinic practice. In clinical teaching, too, students appeared to acquire knowledge with both greater ease and enthusiasm when it was presented in practical, observable settings. In fact, it is this expressed desire for decidedly translatable knowledge—for being able to extract what you read here and apply it to your current or future medical practice—that inspired us to adopt a CBL approach throughout this text.

Why a Case-Based Learning (CBL) Approach

In addition to demonstrating in concrete terms the various facets of healthcare, the introductory case provided above is designed to familiarize you, the reader, with the format of this book, which centers around CBL. CBL, which McLean (2016) defines as "a teaching tool used in a variety of medical fields using human cases to impart relevance and aid in connecting theory to practice" (p. 39), is often considered the gold standard of medical education (Figure 1.2). CBL has proven highly effective for instructing on a wide variety of concepts and topics, from covering the mechanisms behind osteoporosis (Nguyen et al., 2021) to teaching about acute chest syndrome due to sickle cell anemia (Meloy et al., 2023), across all levels of training, making it useful for a first-year medical student just as much as a third-year resident (Fromke et al., 2022). More than holding relevance for diverse groups of learners, though, and as the above definition suggests, the appeal of CBL lies in its emphasis on the practical. CBL demonstrates to the learner how, exactly, the content they are being presented with may show up in their practice. It is this orientation to "real-world" knowledge that inspired us to adopt this particular framework through this book.

In encountering each case presented here, the reader is encouraged to treat the patient featured therein as representing countless previous patients and infinite future ones. These cases thus operate as an amalgam, as a composite of many individuals, and at the same time, no single person at all. While all cases here are hypothetical, they are informed by real clinical encounters, and as such, are meant to be generalizable to a variety of health contexts. In this way, the elements each case is imbued with are designed to resonate with the reader, perhaps not now, but certainly as they travel along their medical education journey.

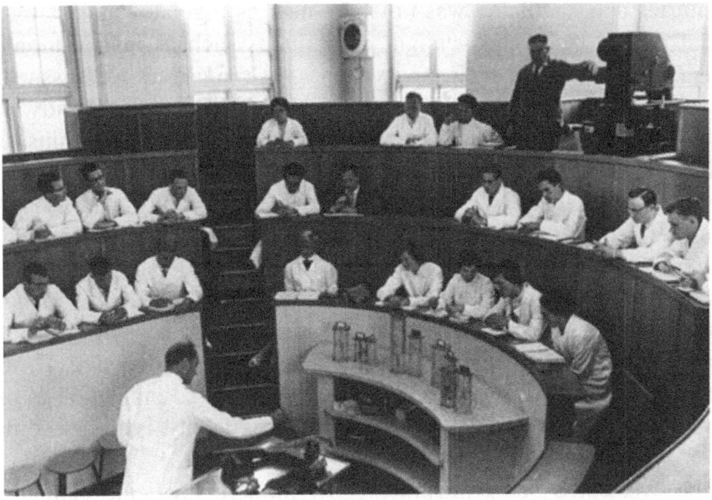

Figure 1.2 Classroom Instruction in Anatomy. Photo from the National Library of Medicine.

Merging Medicine with the Humanities

Having laid out the merits of a CBL approach to medical education, it is now worth examining why one should study the social side of medicine—beyond the anatomical, physiological, and pharmacological learning that practitioners and aspiring practitioners engage with. Studies inquiring into medicine as a social science, in addition to a physical science, are not only justified but also much needed. However, to better understand how social medicine is studied today, it is first necessary to examine how it responds to a centuries-old call for a more *humane* medical practice through the entrance of medical humanities.

The medical humanities are often described as putting the human element back into medicine, leading one to question how it was that humanity was ever missing from medicine in the first place. In his account of how medical humanities as a field of study came to be, Wailoo (2022) describes it as

> a story of growing relevance shaped by tragedy, of innovative programs in medical school and on undergraduate campuses, and vital new configurations of ethics, literature, the arts, and history that breathed new life into the study of health and medicine (p. 194).

Wailoo's claim that the emergence of medical humanities is, in many ways, a response to tragedy points to the fact that the need for this area of study arose from both the historically egregious abuses of medicine and its comparatively more benign instances of overreach in the present day.

Centuries ago, medicine was nowhere near as regulated as it is today—the result of ethical research oversight committees such as **institutional review boards (IRBs)**. Without such supervision, grave injustices were issued against **vulnerable populations**[2] in the name of medical and scientific advancement. One well-known example lies with the case of Dr. J. Marion Simms, often referred to as "the father of modern gynecology." In the mid-19th century, Simms performed experimental gynecological procedures on enslaved Black women without the use of anesthesia, operating on the assumption that Black women had a higher tolerance for pain. In fact, one enslaved woman, Anarcha Westcott, was subjected to more than 30 operations without anesthesia (Ojanuga, 1993). Unfortunately, Westcott's story is just one of many instances in which atrocities were committed under the guise of increasing medical knowledge. The modern-day implications of these violations of the often-touted injunction in medicine to "First Do No Harm"[3] for patients of color, specifically, is discussed further in Chapter 2 (Figure 1.3).

While Westcott's story illustrates how modern medicine benefitted from cruel and exploitative institutions like slavery, such instances of abuse were not confined to the U.S. In Australia in the 1960s and 1970s, vaccine trials were conducted on Aboriginal children who had been forcibly removed from their homes by the state and placed in institutional care (Brady, 2007). These children were not of the age of **consent** (where they could legally agree to participate in a procedure or study), and therefore could not provide it. While they technically

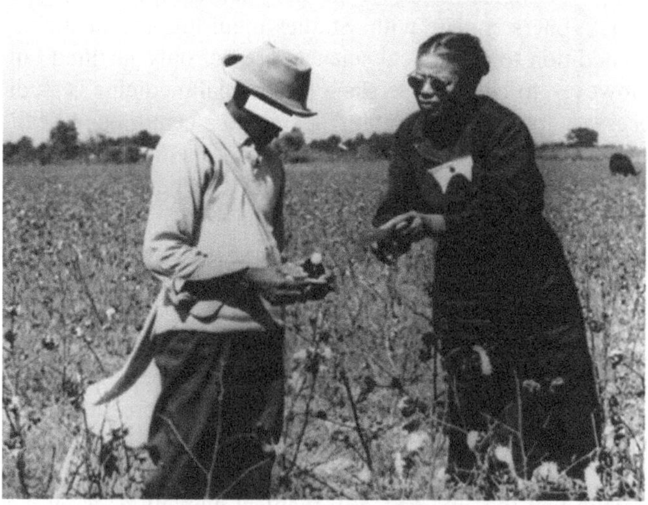

Figure 1.3 Nurse Eunice Rivers visiting a patient in a cotton field in Macon County, Alabama, during the Tuskegee Syphilis Study. Photo from the Centers for Disease Control Public Health Image Library.

could **assent** to participation in the trials (i.e., they could agree to participate, but such agreement would not be considered legally valid due to their status as minors), their legal guardians would need to supply consent. But having been torn from their parental homes, in this case, the state served as their legal guardians, supplying consent on their behalf. The result of these ethical transgressions is a population, many of whom even today are wary of medicine and skeptical that its representatives have their best interest at heart (Kennedy & Bryant, 2024). A similar reluctance toward medicine is likewise observed in the U.S. among some Black patients (refer to Chapter 2 for examples), proving that the injustices committed decades and centuries ago by medical professionals still exert a profound impact on patient well-being in the present day.

Fortunately, at least in the U.S., harmful acts such as those committed by Simms and various federal governments have become less prevalent in the modern era, thanks to legal intervention at the federal level assuming the form of the National Research Act of 1974.[4] Not only did this particular piece of legislation lead to the formation of the first IRBs to ensure that medical research was ethical, but it prompted the creation of the **Belmont Report**. This document outlined three core principles of ethical research, the first of which is **beneficence**. The concept of beneficence echoes the aforementioned injunction to "First, do no harm" by requiring that the research maximizes benefits while minimizing risks for those involved. The second principle, **justice**, states that research populations should be fairly selected, and that benefits should be distributed to all participants, not just those with an already privileged social status. Finally, the third principle, **respect for persons**, requires that an individual fully consent to participation in the research, and that they have done so without coercion or manipulation. In fact, because of the Belmont Report, providers must now ensure that prior to undergoing any procedure, a patient has been thoroughly briefed on both its risks and its benefits.

While the Belmont Report represents the U.S. response to unethical medical practices, there are many international equivalents that both preceded and followed the publication of the report. In fact, as far back as 1947, in the wake of WWII, the scientific community was thinking about how to prevent the forcible experimentation that occurred under the Nazi regime at the behest of Josef Mengele and others. By his hands, and those of his colleagues, Jewish and Roma people, as well as persons with disabilities and countless others, suffered to provide insights into the effects of freezing temperatures and high altitudes on the body (Weindling, 2008). After witnessing these medical crimes, a multinational tribunal developed the Nuremberg Code, which laid the groundwork for several other countries and councils to follow suit. A table detailing the timeline of the development of these documents is presented in Table 1.1.

Despite the significant amount of progress that has been made in ensuring that the transgressions of medical research are never again repeated, there are those who argue that the overreach of medicine occurs in more subtle ways.

Table 1.1 A timeline of international ethical medical research protocols.

Year enacted	*Name of ethical guideline*	*Country involved/ initiated*	*Outcome*
1947	Nuremberg Code	International	The first modern set of codes guiding research ethics, this document emphasized the voluntary nature of consent and asserted that researchers should seek to minimize or eliminate unnecessary harm to participants (Annas & Grodin, 1992).
1964	Declaration of Helsinki	World Medical Association	This document is responsible for establishing the protocol for weighing risks to participants versus benefits, and emphasizes the importance of informed consent (World Medical Association, 2013).
1979	The Belmont Report	United States National Commission for the Protection of Human Subjects of Biomedical and Behavioral Research	The report introduced three core ethical principles for conducting medical research: respect for persons, beneficence, and justice (National Commission, 1979).
1982	International Ethical Guidelines for Biomedical Research Involving Human Subjects	The Council for International Organizations of Medical Sciences (CIOMS), World Health Organization (WHO)	This document provides ethical guidelines for conducting research in developing nations and underresourced areas (CIOMS & WHO, 2002).
1997	Oviedo Convention	Council of Europe	This is a legal treaty touching on human dignity and rights, as well as informed consent within medicine (Council of Europe, 1997).

(*Continued*)

Table 1.1 (Continued)

Year enacted	*Name of ethical guideline*	*Country involved/ initiated*	*Outcome*
1999	Ethics in Health Research: Principles, Structures and Processes	South Africa Department of Health	Provided ethical guidelines following Apartheid and incorporated more diverse cultural values (South Africa Department of Health, 2004).
2001	National Statement on Ethical Conduct in Human Research	Australia's National Health and Medical Research Council	This document aimed to serve the Aboriginal and Torres Straight Islander population with an eye toward justice, beneficence, and research benefit (NHMRC, 2018).
2010	UK Policy Framework for Health and Social Care Research	The United Kingdom Health Research Authority	Provided oversight in all matters related to health research (Health Research Authority, 2017).
2010	National Ethical Guidelines for Biomedical and Health Research Involving Human Participants	Indian Council of Medical Research (2017)	Provides special considerations for the ethics of researching vulnerable/protected populations (ICMR, 2017).
2010	Tri-Council Policy Statement: Ethical Conduct for Research Involving Humans (TCPS 2)	Canadian Institutes of Health Research, Natural Sciences and Engineering Research Council of Canada, & Social Sciences and Humanities Research Council of Canada (2018)	Upholds the principles of respect for persons and justice, but adds guidelines pertaining to Indigenous peoples (TCPS 2, 2018).

Source: Generated by the authors.

These critics contend that the growing presence of medicine in multiple areas of life have led to the "**medicalization**" of society as a whole. One of the most vocal critics of medicalization, Paul Starr (1982), argued that medicine became such a significant source of authority within our society, not just because it improved health outcomes, but because it had the power to define what counted as normal and what counted as illness worthy of medical intervention. Examples of the medicalization of contemporary society are many, and span the gamut of male-pattern baldness to menopause, to acne, to ADHD. Looking specifically at the case of ADHD, what may have once been considered different styles, rates, and approaches to learning is now classified as a medical condition listed in the *Diagnostic and Statistical Manual of Mental Disorders-V (DSM V)* (Forbes, 2015). Scholars like Peter Conrad (2007) argue that even life and death have transformed from normal parts of the human experience into something requiring medical intervention. These events, which happened within the confines of one's own home for most of recorded history, now occur within the hospital walls in most Western settings. To illustrate how recently something like childbirth became a medical phenomenon, scholars often cite the example of former U.S. President Jimmy Carter, who served in office from 1977 to 1981, and was the first U.S. president to be born in a hospital. Prior to then, childbirth occurred at home, relatively outside of medicine proper.

However, one could certainly (and rightly) argue that maternal and infant morbidity and mortality rates have drastically decreased throughout the world due to more medical resources being available to pregnant people. Although there is much merit in this counterpoint critics of medicalization suggest there are more duplicitous motivations behind making more parts of life the concern of medical providers, multinational healthcare systems, and pharmaceutical and medical device manufacturers. These individuals assert that current medical practices are governed by a profit-driven system and that physicians have a professional obligation to act as **stewards** of resources, refraining from the overtreatment of conditions that, perhaps, may not be *conditions* at all.

Narrative Medicine and the Humanization of Medicine

With scholars, practitioners, and even the general public becoming more acutely aware of all that has ailed modern medicine, the stage was thus set for proposing a remedy, and this remedy came in the form of **narrative medicine**. DasGupta (2008) positions narrative medicine orienting to patients' stories not as "objects that we can comprehend or master, but rather dynamic entities that we can approach and engage with, while simultaneously remaining open to their ambiguity and contradiction, and engaging in constant self-evaluation and self-critique" (p. 981). In the past few decades, narrative medicine has gained traction precisely because it resonates with practitioners and patients alike in how it carves out a deliberate space where patients can describe their **chief concern**—the reason for their healthcare visit—in plain language. As the name suggests, storytelling is at the center of *narrative* medicine, with the practice's founder, Rita Charon, describing these stories as supplying what medicine is presently lacking. She describes narrative medicine as "fortifying" clinical practice as a diagnostic tool, one that allows the provider to "recognize, absorb, metabolize, interpret, and be moved by the stories of illness" (p. vii).

Despite the appeal of narrative medicine in its ability to offer patients the opportunity to make sense of their illness on their own terms, it is accompanied by its own set of challenges. For one, narrative medicine is riddled with challenges in implementation. In practicing narrative medicine, Charon advises that clinicians begin each encounter by inviting patients to tell their story, to begin first by saying, "I will be your doctor, so I need to know a great deal about your body, and your health and your life. Please tell me what you think I should know about your situation" (Talesnik, 2019). In theory, this sort of patient-led approach seems very much in line with the ideals of the medical humanities; the problem enters when it comes up against institutional constraints. For example, we saw this in Case 1, where Dr. Nelson is allocated a 20-minute time slot to see a patient who may want to discuss multiple, complex health issues. Inviting the patient to tell their story, uninterrupted, without prompting or guidance from the physician, may therefore present significant concerns for time management in the clinic. Outside of feasibility, there may also be a lack of provider buy-in, especially when many healthcare systems offer financial incentives for productivity, which is often measured in terms of volume (i.e., seeing the most patients in the least amount of time) (Conrad et al., 2002).

That said, while narrative medicine may be considered by some to be largely an ideal, it is nonetheless valuable in how it encourages providers to think about how clinical knowledge may be derived from a variety of sources, patient stories included. At its foundations, narrative medicine prompts providers to ask questions about what constitutes medical knowledge, how it is generated, and who gets to assess its clinical relevance. In fact, what many critics see as a primary disadvantage of narrative medicine—its subjectivity and presumed incompatibility with a scientific model (see Ahlzén, 2019)—others highlight this quality as an inherent advantage. Hurwitz (2000), for example, credits narrative medicine with "enabling clinicians to enter into the subjective world of the patient," where they can "appreciate the moral weight of illness" (p. 49). This is perhaps why narrative medicine has witnessed such profound staying power within the field, as the emphasis it places on the patient's interpretative framework aligns with current understandings of knowledge production as stemming from diverse, and often unexpected, sources.

What a Communication-Based Approach to the Medical Humanities Can Offer

When it comes to knowledge in the clinic, matters are often depicted in black and white: a patient's hemoglobin A1c (HbA1c) comes back as $\geq 6.5\%$, indicating in definitive terms that they have diabetes; human chorionic gonadotropin (β-hCG) is present in the patient's blood, denoting pregnancy; biopsy and immunohistochemistry testing of breast cancer indicate the presence of estrogen receptors. Often, lab results, imaging, and even the findings of a physical exam are regarded as presenting the clinician with objective data points—with factual and indisputable information.

But this is where studies in health communication enter. Scholars of communication have long asserted that all realities, clinical realities included, do not exist independently of the individual perceiving them. They therefore make a distinction between "Truth" with a capital "T" and "truth" with a lowercase "t." The former is meant to signal large-scale assumptions that are taken to be objective and universal, and as not varying according to specific cultural contexts. Big "T" Truths are compatible with a **positivist** philosophical tradition, which assumes that knowledge of different phenomena can be empirically observed or measured and that it can be applied to all people, regardless of the specifics of their individual experiences. An example of such an assumption within medicine may be something as simple as "the human body requires oxygen to live." A fact such as this is clear cut, but there are those that are less so. These clinical realities are more in line with "little t" representations of reality. This approach to knowledge production accounts for how cultural variations, large-scale discourses about different populations or social groups, and the peculiarities of individual experience all influence what someone deems as true or not.

One example of how this shows up in medicine is in the estimation of kidney function in patients of different racial/ethnic backgrounds (Figure 1.4). Historically, this was determined via an estimated glomerular filtration rate (eGFR) equation that was applied differently in Black and Non-Black patient populations. This equation used a lab value called creatinine, a product of muscle metabolism. How quickly an individual can "clear" or remove creatinine from their blood, in the kidneys, is a way of assessing the functional health of that individual's renal system. Until

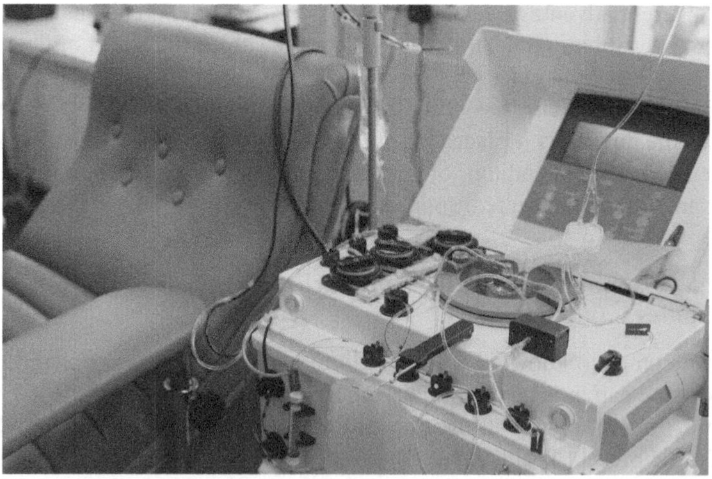

Figure 1.4 A photo of a dialysis machine. Photo from Shutterstock.

guidelines were updated in 2021, a Black patient was given a 16-point-higher eGFR compared to a non-Black patient with the same creatinine levels. This was based on a study by Jones et al (1998). that aimed to improve methods for assessing kidney function using serum creatinine. In the course of their investigation, the researchers discovered that Black patients had higher creatinine levels for the same GFR values when compared to their non-Black counterparts. This observation, in turn, prompted them to recommend a race-adjusted GFR score for Black patients.

The problem is that the recommendations that ensued from these findings were based on a flawed methodological approach. The study itself suffered from significant limitations, most notable of which was its small and non-representative sample, overreliance on race as a biological certainty (to the exclusion of environmental factors), and the inability to forecast the long-term implications of such fundings. The use of the now defunct equation had many clinical implications, such as the false reassurance that individual Black patients had better kidney function than that they may have truly had. Higher doses of renally cleared medications were used to treat this patient population, resulting in higher toxicity levels and greater side effects. Operating on the assumption that Black patients exhibited better renal performance than was actually true resulted in delayed recognition of worsening kidney function, and very likely contributed to the higher rate of chronic kidney disease (CKD) and end-stage renal disease in Black patients (Centers for Disease Control and Prevention, 2023).

As this example shows, seemingly objective data, like numerical values on a lab result, become much less objective when infused with race-based clinical biases. Such biases, in turn, have a direct and significant impact on patient care. If these values are skewed due to adjustment for patient race, and clinicians are basing their treatment recommendations on this information, there is the possibility of delayed diagnosis and subpar CKD management. More than that, one can see how failing to consider how social narratives about different groups of people shape beliefs regarding their care can exacerbate health outcomes that are already disproportionately poor for this vulnerable patient population (Reitman, 2023; Sheikh et al., 2022).

Case 2 presents another instance of how a medical condition that appears to be matter-of-fact for one provider may be differently interpreted for another.

Case 2

Scenario: Mr. Adams is seeing Dr. Price for the first time at an orthopedic office. He has been experiencing several months of atraumatic shoulder pain (Figure 1.5).

Patient: Mr. Adams is a 45-year-old male auto-mechanic with poorly controlled type 2 diabetes (A1c 9.5%). He drinks Coca-Cola during the day to stay hydrated and is sometimes so busy that he forgets his morning metformin dose. He has a 12-year-old daughter that he cares for by himself after his wife died of a narcotic overdose five years ago. His MRI cost him $600 due to his insurance's deductible policy.

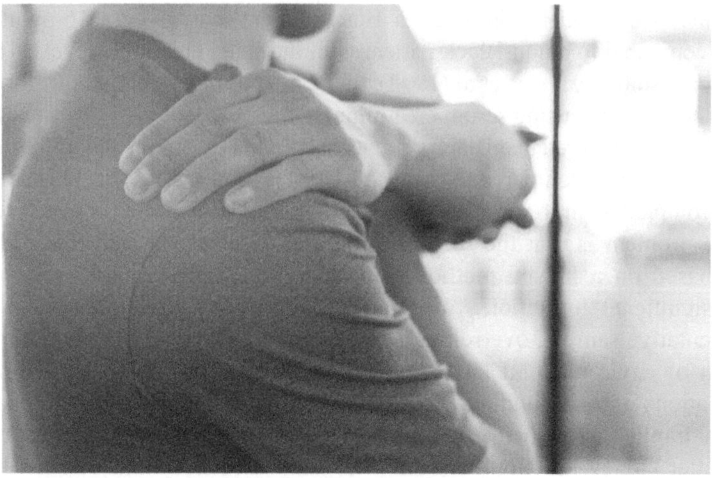

Figure 1.5 A patient with shoulder pain. Photo from Shutterstock.

Providers: Dr. Price is an experienced orthopedic sports medicine surgeon at a private practice. He is accompanied by his medical assistant, Mara, who also acts as a scribe during the encounter. Dr. Cho is Mr. Adams' primary care physician, who has followed Mr. Adams for approximately ten years.

Prior to today's appointment, Mr. Adams requested an MRI at a visit with Dr. Cho. The summary of the MRI report is presented below.

Clinical Summary:

1 Partial-thickness, partial-width, articular sided supraspinatus tear with accompanying low grade, partial-thickness, partial-width tear of the infraspinatus.
2 Moderate degenerative changes of the acromioclavicular joint.
3 Findings suggestive of adhesive capsulitis, including rotator interval edema and axillary pouch thickening.

Mr. Adams reviewed the MRI report with Dr. Cho over the phone. Dr. Cho discussed the findings of the MRI with Mr. Adams, which included a rotator cuff tear and explained what the rotator cuff was. Dr. Cho said that some of his other patients had received arthroscopic surgery for rotator cuff tears and had been able to return to work in about six months. Mr. Adams is relieved to hear that there is a solution to his problems. A coworker also had rotator cuff repair and told him that he is now doing well. With this information, Mr. Adams is looking forward, with some trepidation, to discussing surgery with Dr. Price, as he believes it will fix his shoulder pain so that he can work more comfortably and provide for his daughter.

Dr. Price looks at the images with Mr. Adams, pointing out the rotator cuff tears and the acromioclavicular osteoarthritis on the computer. He also shows him images of edema (swelling) of the rotator cuff interval as well as in the axillary pouch, which are findings of adhesive capsulitis, or frozen shoulder. He then examines Mr. Adams and verbalizes to Mara that there is range of motion loss in all planes of motion of the shoulder, but 5/5 strength on external rotation, internal rotation, and abduction. Ultimately, Dr. Price tells Mr. Adams that arthroscopic shoulder surgery to repair his rotator cuff would not reliably help his symptoms, as Dr. Price thinks they are primarily due to frozen shoulder. Dr. Price suggests improved blood sugar control, physical therapy, and possibly a steroid injection for pain. However, the steroid injection might worsen his blood sugar levels for several days.

The example of Mr. Adams encourages us to think deeply about evidence in medicine—how it is interpreted differently by different parties and acted upon accordingly. The current trend toward **evidence-based medicine (EBM)**, which is now considered the gold standard for medical research and practice, is closely aligned with the principles of a positivist tradition. Simply put, EBM is the "conscientious, explicit, and judicious use of current best evidence in making decisions about the care of individual patients" (Sackett et al., 1996, p. 71). What complicates the decision-making process is that both providers featured here, Dr. Price and Dr. Cho, provide different recommendations using largely the same set of information. Nearly every medical decision is a complex mix of exam findings, patient-reported symptoms, the patient's expressed goals, exam findings, and test results (including labs, images, biopsy results, etc.). Take the example of a blood test. A value that some providers interpret as "borderline" indicative of disease may be regarded as a positive result by others (sedimentation rate, for example). Additionally, while some imaging results may be less ambiguous (i.e., the presence of a fracture on an X-ray), modalities like ultrasound are highly operator-dependent, meaning that the findings may differ based on the individual performing the ultrasound exam and interpreting the images.

In addition to information garnered through exams, tests, and imaging, there is also the information the patient supplies themselves to consider. There is inherent subjectivity in symptom description; a pain scale rating of a "2" for one patient may be a "7" for another.[5] Another point to consider is that patient goals may change over time. At the time of diagnosing rheumatoid arthritis, the patient may express concerns about being able to keep up with their weekly pickleball games. But as their condition worsens, their goals may shift to focus on being able to perform daily tasks, like opening a can or locking a door. Therefore, every aspect of the medical decision-making process is accompanied by some subjective ambiguity.

In Case 2, both providers are acting in accordance with the tenets set forth by EBM in that they are basing their treatment recommendations on the information they have available to them. For Dr. Cho, this information is primarily derived from the MRI report. Dr. Price likewise has this same information accessible to him but is able to supplement it with details obtained through a patient exam and interview. This case illustrates the shift within EBM, which is very much in line with current understandings within communication studies: that meaning is co-constructed between individuals (here, Drs. Cho and Price and Mr. Adams). EBM has largely followed suit with trends in communication studies and now advocates a shared decision-making model of patient care. **Shared decision-making** is a "collaborative process that involves a person and their healthcare professional working together to reach a joint decision about care" (National Institute for Health and Care Excellence, 2021). Rejecting a one-way approach, where providers both tell a patient what is wrong with them and what is best for them, a shared decision-making model of healthcare treats the patient as actively contributing to the meaning of their disease or condition, their preferred treatment plans, and the health outcomes they expect to experience.

In this way, this turn toward shared meaning-making aligns with a broader constructivist view of knowledge in communication theory. Communication theorists adopt a **constructivist approach**, meaning that knowledge of a disease, condition, or illness—and the meaning imparted to it—is not discoverable in the same way that a tumor is, nor is it observable as a chemical reaction. Rather, it is constructed through communication. This approach, when applied in the clinical setting, can be seen in a case where a patient presents with complaints of chronic fatigue, diffuse body aches, and persistent insomnia. Depending on the communicative exchanges between the patient and provider, as well as the provider's interpretive frame, the meaning attributed to the collection of symptoms may simply be chalked up to stress, seen as evidence of a mental health condition like depression, or result in a diagnosis of chronic fatigue syndrome. As Mishler (1984) describes, such meaning-making in medicine involves negotiation between the "voice of medicine"—with its technical, biomedical vocabulary—and the "voice of the lifeworld," which reflects the patient's personal and social experience. All of this is contingent not just upon lab results and physical exams, but upon how well a patient's story aligns with culturally relevant and institutionally sanctioned diagnostic criteria.

The recent emphasis on storytelling, the importance placed on an individual's lived experiences and worldviews in constructing their interpretative frame for making sense of a disease, condition, or constellation of symptoms, and the manner in which providers and patients make sense together all underscore the importance of communication studies to medicine. As those who have witnessed the significance of open, clear, and collaborative communication to clinical interactions firsthand, we have therefore sought to infuse this book on medical education with a distinctly communication-based, humanistic focus. The result, we hope, is not only an educational tool that is supported by current scholarship across disciplines, but one that yields far better patient health outcomes.

Overview of the Chapters

It is because of the integral role of communication within healthcare systems and healthcare encounters that the chapters featured in this book are all oriented around different communication processes relevant to the practice and study of medicine. And consistent with the format and presentation of this chapter, they all employ case studies to illustrate those processes. The following chapter, Chapter 2, is dedicated to exploring intercultural communication and medicine. It looks at the need to account for culturally specific modes of communication via large-scale public health initiatives, for example. On a smaller scale, it considers how culture impacts communication at the level of interaction by examining medicine's historical relationship with members of certain cultures, nationalities, and ethnicities. Within these discussions, we make it a point not to relegate culture to the "exotic," foreign, or other. Rather, in understanding culture as the distinct set of beliefs and practices characterizing a group's way of life and guiding their worldview, we examine co-cultures (previously referred to as "subcultures" within the academic literature) as they exist in relation to the more mainstream dominant culture.

These conversations then set the stage for the topic at focus of Chapter 3: provider and patient positionality. The questions Chapter 3 poses ask how patient and provider identities impact the communication in which they are engaged, and thus the quality of care they receive or provide. Different social identities related to disability, gender, and race or ethnicity will all be addressed here to demonstrate how one's position with society (i.e., their positionality) influences how they make sense of a wide variety of health phenomena. Chapter 3 also attends to the integral role of language in such identity construction work, arguing that within the clinic, seemingly innocuous linguistic choices are highly consequential.

Building off of discussions of the patient-provider concordance that may or may not come with an alignment of social identities and positionalities, Chapter 4 then explores the dual communicative functions of report and rapport. It examines processes and interactions more geared toward information transmission—that is, the report function of communication—as well as exchanges and gestures that work in the interest of rapport-building, which is designed to establish a relationship or connection with the patient. In short, this chapter reflects on rapport-building as both a professional commitment and a diagnostic tool.

Having zoomed out to briefly acknowledge the different parties that may be involved in a healthcare encounter, beyond just the patient and their provider, Chapter 5 expands upon the subject by attending to matters of organizational communication. It inquires into how organizational hierarchies, fixed streams of communication, and the transfer of care impact patient health. Also embedded within this discussion of organizational communication is the topic of organizational culture, as it examines how a hidden curriculum of medicine imparts the tenets of this culture to its professional members.

As a large part of organizational communication occurs through mediated communications, Chapter 6 will be dedicated solely to exploring the role of electronic medical health records in the delivery of care in today's social and technological landscape. This chapter adopts an ethical orientation, inviting questions of artificial intelligence (AI)'s place within medicine, and systematically examining both its potential promises and its perils. It also reflects on how patient portals shape health communication, as now, patients have the ability to directly message their providers with concerns or questions, view lab results as they come in, and read providers' clinical summaries.

Healthcare at the end of life felt like a natural place to close the subject areas introduced in this book on health communication and the medical humanities, and so the last type of communication to be explored here is presented in Chapter 7 on end-of-life communication. This chapter takes a historical approach to the topic of end-of-life care by considering landmark cases in the Right-to-Die movement, and the ethical dilemmas embedded inherent within those. Consistent with this book's communication-based focus, it traces the evolution of the terminology surrounding this movement, and the implications of linguistic choices like "physician-assisted suicide" versus "medical aid in dying." And with a special attention to the medical ethical principles of patient autonomy, justice, non-maleficence, and beneficence, it considers how, in their discussions of end-of-life care, providers may attempt to honor all four.

The final chapter, Chapter 8, questions the future of medicine. It examines current trends in medicine to advocate for a participatory, collaborative, and systemic approach to healthcare delivery. It reflects on how a humanist, communication-forward approach to healthcare might aid in addressing these issues, so that tomorrow's healthcare is effective, just, equitable, and ethical.

Glossary

- **Cross-functional communication**
- **Cognitive load**
- **Emotional labor**
- **Provider burnout**
- **Electronic medical records (EMRs)**
- **Nonverbal communication**
- **Systemic**
- **Institutional Review Boards (IRBs)**
- **Vulnerable populations**
- **Consent**
- **Assent**
- **Belmont Report**

- **Beneficence**
- **Justice**
- **Respect for Persons**
- **Hippocratic Oath**
- **Medicalization**
- **Stewards**
- **Narrative medicine**
- **Chief concern**
- **Positivist**
- **Evidence-Based Medicine (EBM)**
- **Shared decision-making**
- **Constructivist approach**

Discussion Questions

1. Can you think of any example of how society has become "medicalized"?
2. Narrative medicine, while celebrated for its patient-centered focus, is not without its own set of drawbacks. Most of the pitfalls of this practice pertain to feasibility, time constraints, and institutional traditions that value objectivity above all else. How might you leverage the advantages narrative medicine has to offer, while remaining mindful of its relative drawbacks?
3. Scholars like Paul Starr and Peter Conrad argue that medicine has become a pervasive social authority. How might you as a provider be called upon to act in this capacity? What are the ethical implications of this?
4. What does informed consent look like to you? Is it simply a signature on a form? What tangible measures can you take to ensure that your patient fully understands and agrees to the procedure or treatment plan they are about to undergo?
5. Referring to the example of GFR in Black patients, what other examples can you think of where a lab test, imaging, or other medical test may be more subject to interpretation and provider bias?

Activities

1. Thinking back on the example presented in Case 1, visualize all of the communication channels at play in map form. Do some seem busier than others? Are there different junctures where they meet? And in continuing this metaphor of a communication transit system, are there junctures along these highways that are more congested, more prone to break down?
2. For this activity, the class will divide into two teams for a debate. One side will argue the merits of the medicalization of certain conditions. The other side will argue the disadvantages or drawbacks. See if you can come up with other phenomena that may or may not qualify as medical conditions.

Further Reading

- Read about narrative medicine in this foundational article from its pioneer, Rita Charon: Charon, R. (2001). Narrative medicine: a model for empathy, reflection, profession, and trust. *JAMA, 286*(15), 1897–1902.
- Read *The Atlantic*'s take on what qualifies as a medical (psychological condition) and what is just "normal" human affect: https://www.theatlantic.com/ideas/archive/2023/07/anxiety-depression-mental-health-happiness/674728/

Notes

1 In their book *Communicating with Patients*, Silverman et al. (2013) describe nonverbal communication as referring to all aspects of communication other than the use of words. It includes facial expression, eye contact, posture, gesture, tone and pitch of voice, timing of speech, and the physical distance between communicators.

2 The National Commission for the Protection of Human Subjects (1979) defines vulnerable populations as "individuals or groups who, because of their age, mental or physical condition, socioeconomic status, or situational factors, may have diminished autonomy or be at greater risk of being unduly influenced or harmed in research or healthcare settings."

3 While the instruction to "First Do No Harm" is often associated with the Hippocratic Oath, it is mistakenly attributed. In fact, this phrase is actually derived from another one of Hippcrates' works called *Of the Epidemics* (Shmerling, 2020).

4 The National Research Act came as a response to a particularly salient transgression of medical research, one which is etched into the annals of American history: The Tuskegee Syphilis Study. To learn more about this study and implications for clinical practice and medical research in the modern day, turn to Chapter 2.

5 The use of numeric pain scales has been thoroughly problematized within the academic medical literature on the subject (see Baker et al., 2020; Morasco et al., 2018), which has led to the wide-scale adoption of alternative assessment methods, including the now popular FACES model.

References

Ahlzén, R. (2019). Narrativity and medicine: Some critical reflections. *Philosophy, Ethics, and Humanities in Medicine, 14*(1), 9.

American Psychological Association. (2025). *Cognitive load.* https://dictionary.apa.org/cognitive-load

Annas, G. J., & Grodin, M. A. (Eds.). (1992). *The Nazi doctors and the Nuremberg Code: Human rights in human experimentation.* Oxford University Press.

Baker, D. W., O'Connor, M. K., Kessler, L. G., & Sussman, J. B. (2020). Comparison of a pain tolerability question with the numeric rating scale for pain assessment. *JAMA Network Open, 3*(4), e203155. https://doi.org/10.1001/jamanetworkopen.2020.3155

Brady, M. (2007). Equality and difference: Persisting historical themes in health and alcohol policies affecting Indigenous Australians. *Journal of Epidemiology and Community Health, 61*(9), 759–763. https://doi.org/10.1136/jech.2006.057455

Canadian Institutes of Health Research, Natural Sciences and Engineering Research Council of Canada, & Social Sciences and Humanities Research Council of Canada.

(2018). *Tri-Council Policy Statement: Ethical conduct for research involving humans (TCPS 2)*. https://ethics.gc.ca
Centers for Disease Control and Prevention. (2023, November 30). Chronic kidney disease initiative: Data & research. U.S. Department of Health and Human Services. https://www.cdc.gov/kidney-disease/php/data-research/index.html
Conrad, D. A., Sales, A., Liang, S. Y., Chaudhuri, A., Maynard, C., Pieper, L., & Piland, N. (2002). The impact of financial incentives on physician productivity in medical groups. *Health Services Research*, *37*(4), 885–906.
Conrad, P. (2007). *The medicalization of society: On the transformation of human conditions into treatable disorders*. Johns Hopkins University Press.
Council for International Organizations of Medical Sciences, & World Health Organization. (2002). *International ethical guidelines for biomedical research involving humansubjects*. https://cioms.ch/publications/product/international-ethical-guidelines-for-biomedical-research-involving-human-subjects-2/
Council of Europe. (1997). *Convention on human rights and biomedicine (Oviedo Convention)*. https://www.coe.int/en/web/bioethics/oviedo-convention
DasGupta, S. (2008). Narrative humility. *The Lancet*, *371*(9617), 980–981. https://doi.org/10.1016/S0140-6736(08)60440-7
Forbes, S. (2015). Measuring disability: The agency of an attention deficit/hyperactivity disorder diagnostic questionnaire. *Discourse Studies*, *17*(1), 25–40.
Fromke, E. J., Jordan, S. G., & Awan, O. A. (2022). Case-based learning: Its importance in medical student education. *Academic Radiology*, *29*(8), 1284–1286.
Health Research Authority. (2017). *UK policy framework for health and social care research*. https://www.hra.nhs.uk
Hurwitz, B. (2000). Narrative and the practice of medicine. *The Lancet*, 356(9247), 2086–2089. https://www.researchgate.net/profile/Brian-Hurwitz-2/publication/12182857_Narrative_and_the_practice_of_medicine/links/600d5cf145851553a0682672/Narrative-and-the-practice-of-medicine.pdf
Indian Council of Medical Research. (2017). *National ethical guidelines for biomedical and health research involving human participants*. https://ethics.ncdirindia.org/
Jeung, D. Y., Kim, C., & Chang, S. J. (2018). Emotional labor and burnout: A review of the literature. *Yonsei Medical Journal*, *59*(2), 187–193.
Jones, C. A., McQuillan, G. M., Kusek, J. W., Eberhardt, M. S., Herman, W. H., & Coresh, J. (1998). Serum creatinine levels in the US population: Third National Health and Nutrition Examination Survey. *American Journal of Kidney Diseases*, *32*(6), 992–999. https://doi.org/10.1016/S0272-6386(98)70074-5
Kennedy, M., & Bryant, J. (2024). Ethics in Aboriginal and Torres Strait Islander health research: Discussion paper. Lowitja Institute. https://lowitja.org.au/resource/discussion-paper-ethics-in-aboriginal-and-torres-strait-islander-health-research/
McLean, S. F. (2016). Case-based learning and its application in medical and health-care fields: A review of worldwide literature. *Journal of Medical Education and Curricular Development*, *3*, JMECD-S20377.
Meloy, P., Rutz, D. R., & Bhambri, A. (2023). Acute chest syndrome. *Journal of Education & Teaching in Emergency Medicine*, *8*(1), 1–23.
Morasco, B., Lovejoy, T., Hyde, S., Shull, S., & Dobscha, S. (2018). Limitations of pain numeric rating scale scores collected during usual care: Need for enhanced assessment. *The Journal of Pain*, *19*(3), S57–S58.
National Cancer Institute. (2025). Electronic medical record. *NCI Dictionary of Cancer Terms*. https://www.cancer.gov/publications/dictionaries/cancer-terms/def/electronic-medical-rec

National Commission for the Protection of Human Subjects of Biomedical and Behavioral Research. (1979). *The Belmont Report: Ethical principles and guidelines for the protection of human subjects of research.* U.S. Department of Health, Education, and Welfare. https://www.hhs.gov/ohrp/regulations-and-policy/belmont-report/index.html

National Health and Medical Research Council. (2018). *National statement on ethical conduct in human research (Updated 2018)*. https://www.nhmrc.gov.au

National Institute for Health and Care Excellence. (2021). *Shared decision making.* https://www.ncbi.nlm.nih.gov/books/NBK572428/

Nguyen, B., Athauda, G., Kashan, S. B., Weiler, T., & Toonkel, R. L. (2021). Osteoporosis: A small-group case-based learning activity. *MedEdPORTAL, 17*, 11176.

Ojanuga, D. (1993). The medical ethics of the 'father of gynaecology,' Dr J Marion Sims. *Journal of Medical Ethics, 19*(1), 28–31.

Rassolian, M., Peterson, L. E., Fang, B., Knight, H. C., Peabody, M. R., Baxley, E. G., & Mainous, A. G. III (2017). Workplace factors associated with burnout of family physicians. *JAMA Internal Medicine, 177*(7), 1036–1038. https://doi.org/10.1001/jamainternmed.2017.1391

Reitman, E. (2023, July 16). *Yale study documents staggering toll of health disparities for Black Americans.* Yale School of Medicine News. https://medicine.yale.edu/news-article/yale-study-documents-staggering-toll-of-health-disparities-for-black-americans/

Sackett, D. L., Rosenberg, W. M., Gray, J. M., Haynes, R. B., & Richardson, W. S. (1996). Evidence based medicine: What it is and what it isn't. *BMJ, 312*(7023), 71–72.

Sheikh, J., Allotey, J., Kew, T., Fernández-Félix, B. M., Zamora, J., Khalil, A., & van Gelder, M. (2022). Effects of race and ethnicity on perinatal outcomes in high-income and upper-middle-income countries: An individual participant data meta-analysis of 2,198,655 pregnancies. *The Lancet, 400*(10368), 2049–2062.

Shmerling, R. H. (2020, June 22). First, do no harm. *Harvard Health Blog.* https://www.health.harvard.edu/blog/first-do-no-harm-201510138421

Silverman, J., Kurtz, S., & Draper, J. (2013). *Skills for communicating with patients* (3rd ed). CRC Press.

South Africa Department of Health. (2015). Ethics in health research: Principles, processes and structures (2nd ed.). https://knowledgehub.health.gov.za/system/files/elibdownloads/2023-04/NHREC-DoH-2015-Ethics-in-Health-Research-Guidelines-1_0.pdf

Starr, P. (1982). *The social transformation of American medicine: The rise of a sovereign profession and the making of a vast industry.* Basic Books.

Talesnik, D. (2019, November 1). Charon espouses power of narrative medicine. *NIH Record.*

United States. (1974). *National Research Act*, Pub. L. No. 93-348, 88 Stat. 342. https://www.govinfo.gov/content/pkg/STATUTE-88/pdf/STATUTE-88-Pg342.pdf

Wailoo, K. A. (2022). Patients are humans too: The emergence of medical humanities. *Daedalus, 151*(3), 194–212. https://doi.org/10.1162/daed_a_01938

Weindling, P. (2008). *Nazi medicine and the Nuremberg trials: From medical war crimes to informed consent* (Vol. 34). Palgrave Macmillan.

West, C. P., Dyrbye, L. N., & Shanafelt, T. D. (2018). Physician burnout: Contributors, consequences and solutions. *Journal of Internal Medicine, 283*(6), 516–529.

World Medical Association. (2013). World Medical Association Declaration of Helsinki: Ethical principles for medical research involving human subjects. *JAMA, 310*(20), 2191–2194. https://doi.org/10.1001/jama.2013.281053

2 Intercultural Communication in the Clinic and Beyond

Case 1

Scenario: Mrs. Jin Ma is a 78-year-old female who is seen in the emergency department with difficulty breathing, and is eventually admitted (Figure 2.1).

Patient: Mrs. Ma relocated from China three years ago, to live with her adult daughters in Alexandria, Virginia. She is not able to communicate in English. She has a history of stage 3 esophageal cancer, previously treated in China, as well as COPD. She has a 55-year back history of smoking tobacco use.

Providers: Dr. Sanchez-Aguilar, the inpatient hospitalist providing care to Mrs. Ma, is Colombian-American. Dr. Aronson, an American physician of Eastern European descent, serves as the consulting oncologist.

After admission, Mrs. Ma's care team, including Dr. Sanchez-Aguilar and Dr. Aronson, have received the results of her imaging, indicating that her cancer has metastasized to her lungs. Mrs. Ma has consistently declined the use of a translator and wishes that all medical information be delivered to her adult daughters. Since her diagnosis, her daughters have served as her interpreters, with the younger daughter demonstrating better English language proficiency and understanding. The younger daughter also serves as Mrs. Ma's power of attorney and is legally authorized to make medical decisions on her behalf. Upon being updated on her condition, Mrs. Ma's daughter asks the care team not to tell her mother of her cancer diagnosis. She says that she "Doesn't want to ruin her day, and wants her to enjoy the time she has left."

Dr. Sanchez-Aguilar is inclined to honor Mrs. Ma's daughter's request. However, Dr. Aronson strongly disagrees and believes that the diagnosis as well as the prognosis should be shared with Mrs. Ma. Mrs. Ma's admitting nurse, Nurse Smithey, is also concerned about withholding this information from the patient.

From this lone episode, we can glean a great deal about how one's culture (both the provider's and the patient's) influences the nature of the care they receive. First, it points to the fact that, especially within cultures that rely

DOI: 10.4324/9781003654308-2

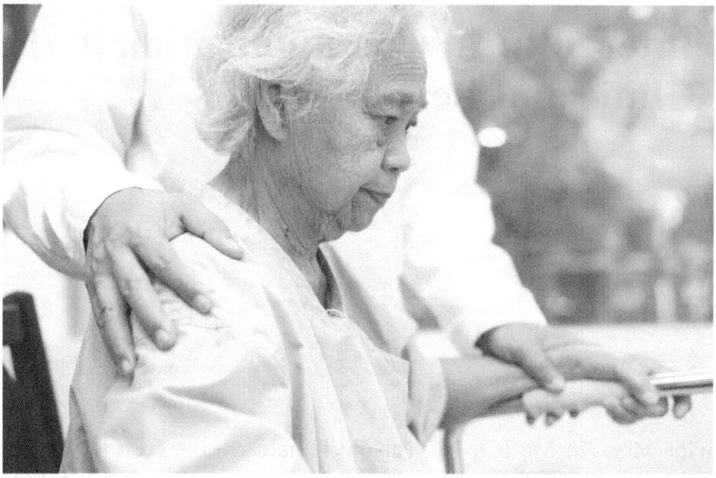

Figure 2.1 An elderly Asian patient uses a walker.

heavily on familial systems and tight-knit social networks, providers will, more often than not, find themselves delivering diagnoses, prognoses, and care plans to more than just the patient. Many Asian societies are characterized by a collectivist culture, wherein matters that affect an individual member of the family are seen as impacting the family unit as a whole. This, coupled with the sense of filial piety that Confucianism endorses (Kyeong et al., 2025), means that the shared decision-making providers typically engage in with patients may now encompass multiple family members. For the provider, this may present several dilemmas. For one, they may find themselves asking about to whom their obligations lie. Must they always act in the patient's best interests, even when those interests run counter to the wishes of the patient's **power of attorney** or designated medical decision-maker? Indeed, providers have a **fiduciary duty** to their patients. As Beauchamp and Childress (1994) explain, "the patient-physician relationship is a fiduciary relationship—that is, founded on trust or confidence; and the physician is therefore necessarily a trustee for the patient's medical welfare" (p. 430). However, don't providers also have an obligation to demonstrate cultural sensitivity? More importantly, what happens when their ethical and perhaps legal duties (here, the obligation to inform the patient of their own condition) are in opposition to the patient's cultural values?

Questions such as these are the impetus behind this chapter on intercultural communication in healthcare settings. As the above case demonstrates, one can see how culture has a direct and inseparable bearing on the nature of communication that unfolds between the provider and those they are caring for. Engaging with these sorts of questions has become more important than ever before, as the world becomes more globalized and individual countries more diverse. In the U.K., data from the 2021 census conducted by the Office for National Statistics (ONS) (2022) supports this claim, indicating that 16.8% of the residents in England and Wales were foreign born (approximately 10 million people). Canada possesses an equally diverse population, with 2021 census data identifying 23% of the country's population, or 8 million people, as being born outside of the country (Statistics Canada, 2022). And while the number of immigrants residing in the U.S. makes up a comparatively lower proportion of the entire population at 13.9%, the number of individuals hailing from a culture that is not American amounts to a sizable 46 million (U.S. Census Bureau, 2024). In light of these figures, the need for greater cultural competency is clear. (For a visualization of these demographic trends by country, see Figure 2.2.)

This chapter begins by introducing a case that encourages providers to think about how culture and family dynamics affect communication preferences and the delivery of care. It reflects not only on how patients' cultures enter the picture, but how providers' do as well. Case 2 then presents culture not as an obstacle to be overcome within the clinic, but as a frame of reference providers can

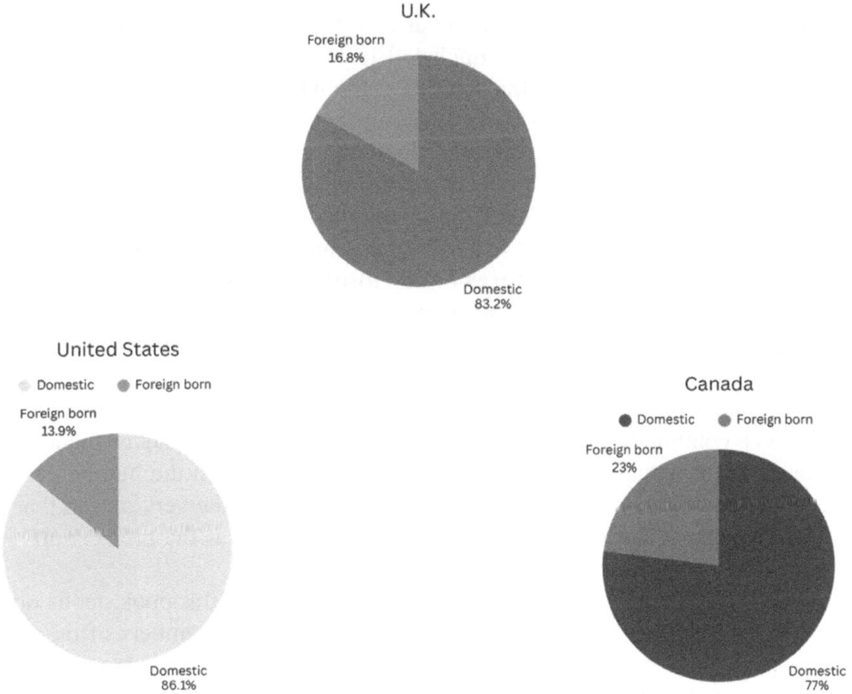

Figure 2.2 A side-by-side comparison of national population composition. Figure was author-generated.

work within to help patients achieve their health goals. After introducing the merits of a culturally sensitive approach, Case 3 prompts healthcare professionals to consider when culture works against the patient's health and well-being. Finally, Case 4 closes out the discussion of culture by encouraging clinicians to conceive of it not as something exotic, foreign, or "other," but as local, regional, and entirely familiar.

Culture, Concordance, and Clinical Care

"Culture" has been defined as "a shared system of values, beliefs, and learned patterns of behavior" (Bigby, 2003, p. 2). In many ways, medical education programs would meet this definition of culture, as they are complete with their own set of rituals, traditions, and even languages. Take the infamous white coat ceremony that marks the culmination of medical school training. Medical students throughout the world participate in this symbolic ritual, wherein they receive their first white coat. This typically occurs early during their first year in medical school, and is accompanied by the reading of a modified version of the Hippocratic Oath. While the white coat is usually shorter than those worn by graduated physicians, the ceremony serves as a type of initiation ceremony into the practice of medicine. The coat is a marker of their membership but also a reminder that they have much left to learn (see Chapter 4 for a more extensive discussion of how the symbol of the white coat functions as a communicative tool).

As this example shows, "culture" does not exclusively refer to the unfamiliar. This chapter therefore makes a point to include more global examples of culture, as well as more localized or regional instances. We do this in acknowledgment of the fact that within virtually any given community, there are bound to be countless **subcultures** or **co-cultures**. Subcultures have traditionally defined themselves as in opposition to the mainstream or dominant culture. Examples include punk, hip hop, gaming, and body modification (e.g., tattoos and piercings) cultures, to name a few. **Co-cultures**, however, are seen as co-existing alongside the mainstream cultures; representative examples include the LGBTQ+ community, the Deaf community,[1] and many immigrant communities, among others. Within the field of communication studies and the humanities in general, "co-culture" has become the preferred term, for the very reason that it does not suggest that one culture is superior to another, as the prefix "sub" in "subculture" might suggest.

Keeping in line with the communication orientation of this book, let us now turn to the language of medical discourse that nearly all members of the care team, from nursing assistants to technicians, learn to adopt. In this shared system of meaning, a "heart attack" becomes a "myocardial infarction," "heartburn" becomes "gastric reflux," and "runner's knee" becomes "patellofemoral syndrome." Your ability to effectively navigate the culture of your nursing program or your medical school requires a thorough understanding of the cultural dynamics of these communities, what is often referred to as "cultural competence."

"**Cultural competence**" has been described as the "ability of health care professionals to communicate with and effectively provide high-quality care to patients from diverse sociocultural backgrounds" (Betancourt & Green, 2010, p. 583). Given the changing national demographics referenced above, healthcare providers have an unprecedented need to be culturally competent. Case 1 also highlights how **patient-provider concordance** (or the lack thereof) bears down on the healthcare interaction. "Concordance," in this case, refers to the degree of alignment between a provider's health beliefs and values and a patient's. Health beliefs and values, though, are inherently shaped by one's cultural background. For this reason, when a provider and a patient come from different cultural backgrounds, a lesser degree of patient-provider concordance is likely—that is, unless the provider is sufficiently culturally competent.

Patient-provider concordance has been discussed at length within the academic literature on the subject, specifically as it relates to improved health outcomes. Saha et al.'s (1999) study of the responses from the 1994 Commonwealth Fund's Minority Health Survey found that Black patients whose care was overseen by Black physicians were more likely to rate their physicians as excellent. Along these same lines, Latin patients receiving care from Latin providers were more likely than those with non-Hispanic physicians to be "very satisfied" with the care they received. More than just leading to improved patient satisfaction, though, patient-provider concordance has been shown to result in improved health outcomes. In Francophone Canada, for example, Reaume et al. (2025) found that when there was a linguistic concordance between providers and allophone patients (i.e., patients whose primary language was neither English nor French), they were at a 36% lower risk of experiencing a major adverse cardiovascular event.

But "concordance" suggests that there is an alignment between *two or more* elements. In the case above, we made it a point to provide information regarding the cultural backgrounds of Mrs. Ma's care team. This was done for several reasons, the first of which seeks to avoid treating Western culture as the default for all clinical care interactions. It is important to note that providers, as well as patients, bring with them their own set of beliefs and values—many culturally laden, others derived from alternative sources of influence like family systems and their own healthcare experiences. Therefore, it is not just the patient's culture that impacts care, but the provider's as well. We learn from the case details provided above about members of the care team's own unique cultural backgrounds, suggesting that these individual-specific characteristics should be accounted for in attempting to reconcile Mrs. Ma's health, her family's wishes, and the standards of care in this episode.

We also chose to include descriptions of the providers' cultural backgrounds in a way that realistically reflected an increasingly diverse health workforce.

The profile of students matriculating into medical school does well to illustrate this point. The Association of American Medical Colleges (AAMC) reported that for the 2023–2024 academic year, enrollment figures for Black students was 10%, up from 8.4% in 2016–2017. Students of Hispanic origin represented 12.7% of enrollees, compared with 10.5% in 2016–2017. These trends furthermore are not limited to a specific national context or professional role. In the U.K., there has also been an increase in the diversity of the composition of the healthcare workforce, with the NHS Workforce Race Equality Standard report indicating that Asian, Black, and other minority ethnic staff constituted over a quarter (25.7%) of the health workforce in 2022, compared with 15.9% in 2009 (NHS, 2025).

Culture as the Communication Context

These figures bode well for patient health, given the findings regarding patient-provider concordance reported above. That said, it is not always feasible to ensure that the provider and patient derive from similar cultural backgrounds. Take the example of the following patient—a 52-year-old male originally from Mexico City, now living in Toronto, with a near-native level of English language proficiency (Figure 2.3). The provider has asked him to report the severity of his abdominal pain. The patient is doubled over, wincing, profusely sweating, and repeatedly vomiting, yet reports their pain to be "not very severe." A culturally competent provider well-versed in the concept of **machismo**, which is prevalent in many Latin cultures and ties cultural notions of masculinity to physical

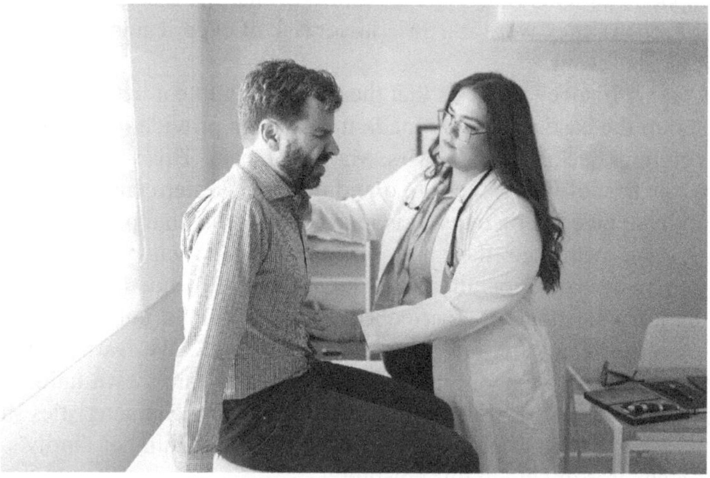

Figure 2.3 A physician performs an abdominal exam on a patient who winces with pain. Photo from Shutterstock.

strength, may gently pursue the veracity of this self-reported assessment. However, with this example, it is important to note that while machismo may play a central role in many Latin cultures, it is not universally relevant. Some countries like Costa Rica and Uruguay, for example, have made marked progress toward promoting gender equality, thus undermining the salience of machismo in the process (World Economic Forum, 2023). Therefore, while it may benefit providers to familiarize themselves with culturally specific beliefs, concepts, and practices, they nonetheless want to refrain from treating Latin, Asian, or any other culture as a monolith.

Indeed, part of what makes one culturally competent is being able to fully grasp the nuances of cultural differences and how those enter into the clinical space. In Mrs. Ma's case, being culturally competent may look like understanding that the family's desire to withhold vital health information from the patient is a common practice in many—though again, not all—Eastern cultures. In Japan, up until as recently as the 1980s, it was commonplace for providers to withhold health information regarding cancer diagnoses and poor prognoses from patients (Powell, 2006). Similar practices have likewise prevailed in China throughout the ages. In their article featured in the *AMA Journal of Ethics*, Nie (2012) acknowledges that "medical professionals in China (including Hong Kong and Taiwan) routinely withhold information about terminal illness from patients, usually inform family members only, and sometimes along with relatives even lie to patients" (p. 243). To better understand why this practice has taken hold in the East but not in the West, one must first examine culturally rooted communication styles, which, as Mrs. Ma's case suggests, are not always compatible with information disclosure in a Western healthcare setting.

The field of communication studies distinguishes between cultures that exhibit **high-context communication**, and those that engage in communication styles that may be considered low-context. **Low-context communication** is, by and large, direct and explicit. This communication style is typical throughout the Global North, particularly in the U.S., Canada, the U.K., Germany, and Scandinavia. With high-context communication, however, there is an emphasis on allowing the parties in communication with one another to save face (i.e., to avoid embarrassment), act politely, and maintain the harmony of the relationship. In fact, the focus on communicating in a way that allows harmonious group dynamics to be upheld is why this mode of communication is found throughout collectivist cultures, like Japan, Korea, and China, where the overall well-being of the society is often prized above individual desires. Case 1 illustrates how the high-context nature of communication styles prevalent in Eastern cultures enter into the clinical space. In an effort to preserve the harmony both within their immediate family, as well as within their interactions with the healthcare team, Mrs. Ma's daughters request that negative information related to her diagnosis and prognosis be withheld from her. In doing so, they are presumably attempting to allow Mrs. Ma to avoid the potential embarrassment that may accompany an emotional reaction to such news.

As the name suggests, high-context communication is highly dependent on the surrounding context of the encounter. Rather than be stated outright, meaning is implied, and often conveyed through the subtleties of body language, facial expressions, and other nonverbal cues. So then, what are the implications of this culturally specific means of communication for providers? Consider the example of informed consent. Current guidelines for obtaining informed consent to participate in research or undergo a procedure must be overt. Both the Declaration of Helsinki (World Medical Association, 2013) and U.S. federal regulations established by the Department of Health and Human Services (2009) emphasize the need for consent to be explicit, and so strongly urge researchers and clinicians to obtain written consent from participants/patients. Let's imagine that Mrs. Ma is eligible to participate in a clinical trial for a drug that may improve her prognosis. In light of cultural styles of communication that prioritize a high-context mode of delivery, she may believe that her wishes to participate in the trial or not are implicitly understood by members of the care team, when in fact, they are not. We can see how, without overt, documented consent, this may not only lead to communication breakdowns but also invite ethical and legal issues to arise.

Outside of communication styles, language also makes up a large part of culture. The practice of family members serving as ad hoc interpreters is widespread throughout medicine. The reasons for patients preferring family members to fulfill this role, as opposed to an institutionally appointed interpreters, are many. Some of the most frequently cited reasons, however, include availability as hospitals and clinics often do not have interpreters on staff at all times (Jaeger et al., 2019), especially for less commonly spoken languages; a distrust of institutions like the medical institution (refer to Chapter 1 and the end of this chapter for a more detailed discussion of the reasons for this distrust); an understanding of cultural norms as opposed to mere linguistic proficiency; and finally, trust in and emotional connection with the interpreter/family member (Hadziabdic et al., 2014). The last of these reasons is a primary reason why patients frequently enlist the help of a family member to interpret on their behalf. They regard their family members as more than mere translators, but patient advocates responsible for promoting their best interest.

Having a family member serve in lieu of a professional medical interpreter, however, raises several ethical and practical concerns. One of these is that the responsibility of interpreting such highly consequential information may place an undue burden on the family member, leading to heightened emotional distress, especially among minors and children performing this role (Pandya, 2023). Other concerns that often appear within the literature on the subject include the possibility for coercion if a family member chooses to interpret information according to their own interests rather than the patient's. Moreover, from the perspective of the patient's health outcomes, when family members assume the role of interpreter, they risk inaccurate or incomplete translation of health information due to a lack of familiarity with medical terminology and discourse. If this information is not properly relayed to the patient, they are unable to participate in truly informed decision-making.

Tittley et al. (2024) examined the dilemma of seeking linguistic and cultural concordance using informal interpretation services within a nursing context. In their study of nurses and nurse practitioners in Ontario, Canada, the authors found that in the face of a lack of institutional support, the providers featured in the study often resorted to flexible workarounds to overcome linguistic and cultural barriers. These workarounds included relying on untrained interpreters like family members, using technological assistance such as Google Translate, resorting to nonverbal communication, scheduling patients only when interpreters were available, and accepting only partial understanding. While the practitioners in this study can be praised for their adaptiveness and ingenuity amidst a lack of institutional resources and support, the study highlights the potential negative implications of these practices with respect to informed consent protocols, clinical accuracy, and patient safety.

As this particular study shows, there are certainly merits to providers pursuing innovative problem-solving methods to bridge cultural and linguistic divides. However, our labeling of these practices as workarounds may be misleading, as what we seek to do is work *within* culture rather around it. Case 2 explores this concept in greater depth.

Working within Culture

Case 2

Scenario: Mrs. Diya Chatterjee is seen at a surgery (outpatient clinic) in London for a consultation regarding atraumatic, left plantar foot pain. Dr. Tariq is seeing Mrs. Chatterjee.

Patient: Mrs. Chatterjee is a 45-year-old computer programmer who works from home. She has had the pain for several months, and it is typically worse in the morning. She walks after work in a nearby park with her husband after work, nightly. Additionally, she follows a vegetarian diet.

Provider: Dr. Tariq, a female general practitioner (GP), is returning from a house call with another patient. This is her first position after completing her medical training.

As Dr. Tariq talks with and examines Mrs. Chatterjee, she suspects that her foot pain is due to plantar fasciitis (Figure 2.4). Dr. Tariq recommends changing to a newer pair of shoes, trying a week of scheduled ibuprofen, and provides a

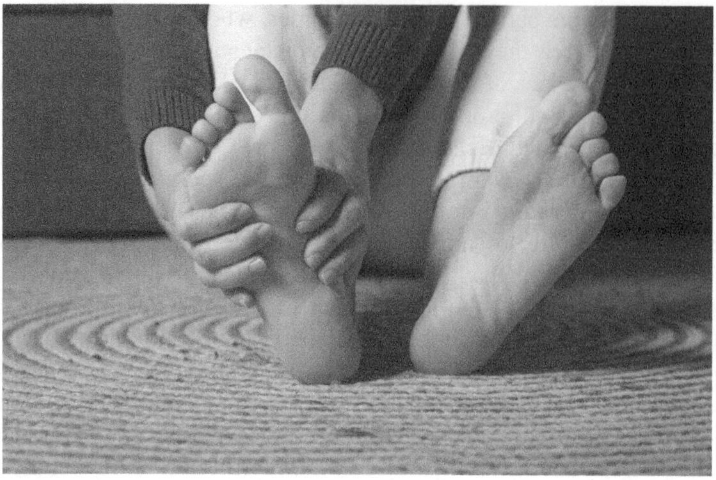

Figure 2.4 A woman grabs the underside of her foot, consistent with plantar fasciitis. Photo obtained from Shutterstock.

home exercise program. Mrs. Chatterjee asks if her vegetarian diet contributed to her foot injury, specifically if she is B12 deficient or lacks sufficient calcium.

Dr. Tariq asks Mrs. Chatterjee about what she eats in a typical day, but nonetheless states that plantar fasciitis is not caused by vitamin or nutrient deficiency. She states that some medical conditions are related to dietary practices that can be mitigated by appropriate supplementation. However, plantar fasciitis is not one of these conditions. Mrs. Chatterjee then asks for recommendations about appropriate supplements and whether she should be tested for any deficiencies.

One of the key takeaways from this encounter is that providers can demonstrate cultural competency by remaining sensitive to specific cultural practices while at the same time providing sound medical advice. They do this by working *within* culture instead of around it. While Dr. Tariq is careful to dispel any misconceptions regarding the impact of a vegetarian diet on musculoskeletal health, she also does not want to come across as dismissing her patient's concerns. Dr. Tariq inquires about what the patient typically eats in order to identify opportunities to incorporate sources of B12 into her diet while nonetheless valuing culturally specific dietary preferences.

Such an approach holds valuable applications to other instances wherein a provider may find themselves engaged in nutrition counseling. The WHO cites obesity as a growing global health concern, with 2022 figures placing 43% of the world population as being overweight and 16% as obese (WHO, 2025). The organization furthermore notes that this epidemic is especially pronounced in the Americas, where, as noted earlier in this chapter, societal demographics are quite diverse. Part of the problem behind these figures may be a misalignment between current medical recommendations for weight loss and cultural cuisine and cooking methods. Let's say that a patient comes from the American South, where the cuisine is high in calories, saturated fats, sodium, and carbohydrates. This patient comes to their provider looking for weight loss options that do not involve medications that their insurance does not cover (and that they can thus not afford) like GLP-1s. The provider may, like Dr. Tariq does above, ask the patient to walk them through what they typically eat. Imagining that the patient recounts fare traditionally associated with this region and culture—breaded chicken deep-fried in oil or lard, collard greens cooked in animal fat, macaroni and cheese, cornbread, and candied yams (sweet potatoes topped with brown sugar, butter, and nuts)—the provider may be able to offer healthier alternatives. Instead of deep-frying the chicken, might they consider grilling it or air frying it? And instead of using animal fat to cook the greens, why not try coconut oil? Offering suggestions such as these can provide an avenue for the patient to achieve their health goals while still respecting cultural traditions. Perhaps more importantly, though, is the fact that encouraging patients to make manageable changes to their eating habits, and ones that are compatible with their cultural traditions, helps to ensure that the effects of these changes are sustainable long-term.

In the case of Mrs. Chatterjee, however, it is also important to point out that the degree of **acculturation** she has experienced may impact her health beliefs. The Stanford Geriatric Education Center (n.d.) defines acculturation in the following manner:

> Acculturation can be defined as a continuum. At one end, the retention of values and beliefs from one's own culture of origin is maintained. Moving towards the center of the continuum, one can become bilingual and bicultural, easily shifting from traditional practices to adopting practices of the mainstream society. At the end of the continuum, individuals may fully adopt the values and beliefs of mainstream society, thus no longer identifying with their original culture.

With this definition in mind, then, Dr. Tariq would be wise to reflect on where Mrs. Chatterjee falls along this continuum. Since she has resided in the U.K. for a considerable amount of time, she may be more knowledgeable of Western cultural practices, and may therefore be more willing to incorporate them into her existing cultural framework. For her, this may not involve incorporating burgers or meatloaf into her diet, but she may be willing to integrate vegetarian options that are not traditionally associated with Indian cuisine, but are routinely available within a Western cultural setting. Dr. Tariq can thus propose that Mrs. Chatterjee supplement her diet with fortified cereals or plant-based milks, add nutritional yeast to her dishes, or turn to fortified meat substitutes to obtain B12. Alternatively, she may wish to consider adding a B12 supplement to her daily regimen. These suggestions may be more palatable to someone like Mrs. Chatterjee, who has lived in the U.K. for an extended period of time, or a second-generation immigrant born in the country, than an individual who is newly arrived.

Turning now to a non-Western health context, Collins Airhihenbuwa has dedicated much of his work to examining how Western medical professionals may inadvertently displace or devalue local health beliefs. Looking specifically at the care provided throughout the African continent, Airhihenbuwa (1990) developed his PEN-3 model, part of which involves classifying health beliefs as positive, existential, or negative. Positive health beliefs are ones that are culturally rooted and exert a beneficial health impact, and should thus be encouraged. Breastfeeding infants may represent a positive health belief to be encouraged, especially in areas where clean drinking water is not readily accessible. Existential health beliefs are neutral—they will neither harm the patient's health, nor help it. An example would be the belief associated with traditional Chinese medicine that drinking cold beverages (e.g., ice water) disrupts one's Qi (lifeforce energy) (Kaptchuk, 1986). Because this health belief does not pose an imminent threat to patient well-being, there is no need for the health provider to "correct" it. In fact, if one were to do so, this could be seen as both **ethnocentric** and **paternalistic**. Put simply, "ethnocentrism" refers to "the belief or attitude that one's own cultural view is the only correct cultural view" (Stanford Medicine, 2019). Paternalism in medicine, however, is the notion that the medical professional "knows best." Under a paternalistic framework, they operate as a parent-like figure (i.e., paternal), and the patient is deemed childlike, devoid of agency. The two constructs often come together within medicine when providers attempt to overlay their cultural beliefs on top of the patient's in order to get them to adopt a particular course of action without an evidence-based reason to do so.

For an example of ethnocentrism gone wrong in a public health context, one only has to look as far as the 2014 Ebola outbreak in West Africa. Public health campaigns were largely seen as failing to curb the spread of the virus due to a pronounced lack of cultural competency. For one, officials neglected to account for the widespread cultural practice of washing dead bodies as a funeral rite (Fairhead, 2016). Simply instructing individuals to "not touch dead bodies" failed to stem the spread of the virus because epidemiological realities could not override centuries-old cultural traditions (Figure 2.5). Furthermore, and on the subject of traditions, many of the regional cultures throughout West Africa were based in an oral tradition, meaning that information was primarily conveyed through spoken word. As a result, text-based campaigns involving posters or other visual messaging systems did little to encourage the public's buy-in (Bedrosian et al., 2016). Finally, a legacy of colonialism resulting in a distrust of outside forces dictating social protocols also played a key role in the ineffectiveness of these

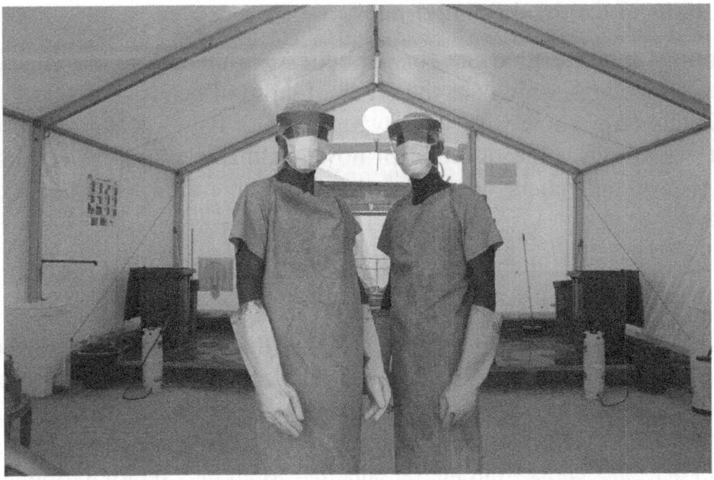

Figure 2.5 A burial team in Sierra Leone dons hazmat suits during the Ebola outbreak. Photo from Shutterstock.

public health interventions (Pellecchia et al., 2015). The Ebola outbreak underscores not only the importance of culturally competent medicine, but also the need to identify which cultural beliefs work in service of health goals and which work against them.

Additionally, views on paternalism have shifted dramatically within just a few generations in Western societies. Previously, healthcare was focused on the absence of illness and on treatment for conditions once they arose. Providers, particularly physicians, were perceived as the sole experts of disease diagnosis and arbiters of appropriate treatment. Gradually over several generations, this gave way to increasing openness of "non-traditional" medical care, focused more on mental health, prevention of disease, diet, exercise, and non-Western views, such as the Qi mentioned above. Further altering the global healthcare landscape is that those seeking or receiving medical care are increasingly viewed as consumers of healthcare. With increasing information available online, providers caring for younger patients are increasingly challenged to explain their thought processes and why or why not certain labs or imaging ordered, or treatments offered. Thus, providers may feel pressed to provide the expected paternalistic care to an older patient, while the next patient from a younger generation may come in with AI-generated diagnosis and holistic treatment plan for the provider to implement (see Chapter 6 for a further discussion of AI, paternalism, and patient autonomy). In this way, we are reminded that culture is not a static social phenomenon, but one that evolves according to generational preferences for care and even the technologies available to providers.

The Limits of Cultural Relativism

This brings us to the final category of beliefs Airhihenbuwa introduces, negative health beliefs, which are the types of cultural beliefs that stand to harm individuals or public health. This type of health belief is at work in Case 3, a case which poses the question of how healthcare providers can intervene so as to promote patient welfare while at the same time remaining culturally sensitive.

Case 3

Scenario: Pediatric Nurse Practitioner (N.P.) Allison Godfrey is seeing her nine-year-old patient, Asha. Asha has been under N.P. Godfrey's care since she was 5. Today, she is performing her annual exam, so N.P. Godfrey looks for signs of sexual development and inquires about Asha's impending puberty with her. She learns from her parents that when they return to Somalia, they plan to have a circumcision performed on her.

Patient: Asha is a nine-year-old girl originally from Somalia, who recently immigrated to Minneapolis, Minnesota (USA). She and her family are practicing Muslims, and heavily involved in their local religious community (Figure 2.6).

Provider: N.P. Godfrey is a Minnesota native and has been practicing in her current pediatric clinic for eight years. Given Minneapolis' large population of Somali immigrants, a significant number of the patients she sees are of this ethnic and national background.

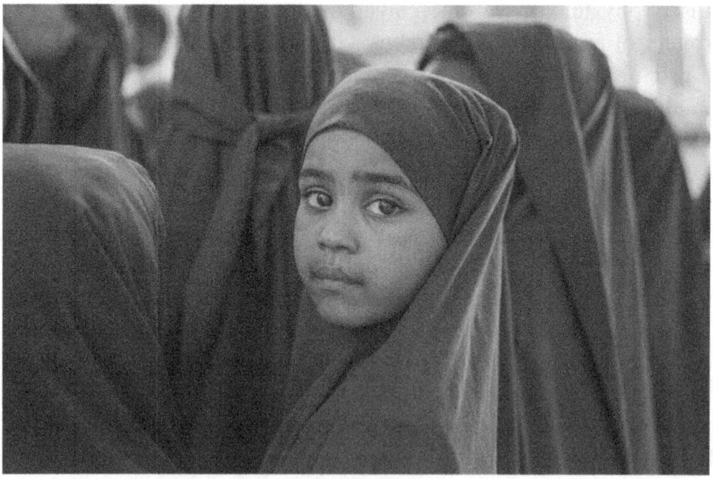

Figure 2.6 A young girl wearing a hijab. Photo obtained from Shutterstock.

This brief episode illustrates several concepts germane to the discussion at hand. The first of these pertains to cultural relativism, and the shortcomings therein. **Cultural relativism**, according to the British Medical Association (2024), "is the position that an act is right or wrong in so far as it is right or wrong for a particular culture." On the one hand, there are those who may argue that in light of the tenets put forth by cultural relativism, if the healthcare provider were to intervene by contacting Child Protective Services or other relevant child welfare agency, such would be an act of ethnocentrism because the practice is not viewed as immoral or unethical within the context of some Somali cultures. However, there are those who adopt a universalist position that advocates that there are certain fundamental human rights, such as those established by the United Nations' (1948) Declaration of Human Rights, that must be upheld no matter what. For them, culture cannot excuse violations of these rights.

The debate over the extent of the protections afforded by culture in this case is moreover reflected in the language used to describe this specific cultural practice. Proponents of the culturally relative position often favor the more neutral "female genital circumcision" in an attempt to destigmatize the practice, and even to draw parallels to the practice of male infant circumcisions (Earp, 2014), which is commonplace in the U.S., Israel, and throughout many Muslim-majority countries. Other more neutral alternatives that have been used to describe this practice include "female genital alteration," which seeks to similarly remove evaluations of the practice from its wording (Shell-Duncan & Hernlund, 2000; Sundby et al., 2013).

Opponents of the practice, on the other hand, endorse the more loaded "female genital mutilation" precisely because it draws attention to the extreme harm the practice imparts. This is the terminology the United Nations Population Fund (2025) employs, as the organization states that this wording "more accurately describes this practice from a human rights viewpoint." So, then, what language should N.P. Godfrey use in her conversations with the patient and her parents? In the context of other decisions surrounding language in the clinic (see Chapter 3 for further details), most clinicians and scholars advocate a patient-led or **patient-matched** approach (Williams & Ogden, 2004). This means that N.P. Godfrey should use the language that the patient and her family do. Opting instead for "female genital mutilation" may shut down the conversation with the patient and her parents as it implies judgment and may even suggest condemnation. By keeping the conversation going in this way, N.P. Godfrey is afforded the opportunity to educate the patient and her family about the serious health risks posed by this practice, which range from infection to childbirth complications that result in higher maternal and infant mortality rates (World Health Organization, 2023). If the family, however, is steadfast in their decision, N.P. Godfrey might practice **harm reduction**, which involves seeking to minimize the harm imposed by a health behavior without necessarily eliminating it. A classic example of harm reduction include programs designed to provide clean hypodermic needles to intravenous drug users. The logic behind these initiatives acknowledges that immediately preventing drug use may not be feasible under all circumstances; however, preventing the blood-borne diseases (e.g., HIV and hepatitis C) that are spread through used needles may be obtainable through syringe supply programs (National Harm Reduction Coalition, 2024). N.P. Godfrey could apply a similar rationale here, and practice harm reduction by advising the family to have the procedure performed by a medical professional or in a sterile environment rather than by a traditional community exciser. It is worth noting, however, that the WHO (2025) discourages medicalizing the practice in this way, as it may inadvertently legitimize it.

One last option available to N.P. Godfrey is to enlist the help of community leaders in encouraging **patient adherence** (here, patient and family adherence). The WHO (2003) defines patient adherence as "the extent to which a person's behaviour-taking medication, following a diet and/or executing lifestyle changes, corresponds with agreed recommendations from a healthcare provider." Patient adherence represents the preferred terminology over its predecessor "**patient compliance**," which some have argued reflects medicine's historically paternalistic approach to patient care and the implicit assumption that patients will passively follow providers' orders (i.e., they will *comply*). Within the context of this example, patient adherence would look like the patient and her family choosing to forego the planned procedure due to the significant health risks it imposes. In order to encourage such adherence, and recognizing that different patient populations may demonstrate various degrees of skepticism toward the medical institution and its representatives, N.P. Godfrey may encourage the family to contact an imam or other spiritual leader within the local Muslim community. This individual could help clarify that this practice has no religious basis in the Islamic faith, and thus persuade the family to abandon their plans. But more than soliciting the help of the community leader to dispel any misconceptions that tie the practice to a particular religious belief, this individual may be able to serve as a liaison between this patient population and the medical institution, effectively brokering trust where it has been historically lacking.

When it comes to fostering patient adherence, tapping community leaders in this way has a proven track record of success. In campaigns designed to encourage patient adherence to HIV treatment in Sub-Saharan Africa, public health officials sought the help of religious leaders (primarily pastors and imams) to destigmatize both the disease and the antiretroviral (ART) therapies associated with it. The religious leaders at the center of this campaign incorporated overt support for ART in their sermons, offered basic health education, and even paid members of their community home visits to help ensure adherence (Alio et al., 2019).

Another example of engaging community leaders for the betterment of public health is the often-cited "Barbershop Study" (Victor et al., 2018) (Figure 2.7). The study followed 319 Black male patrons of 52 barbershops throughout the

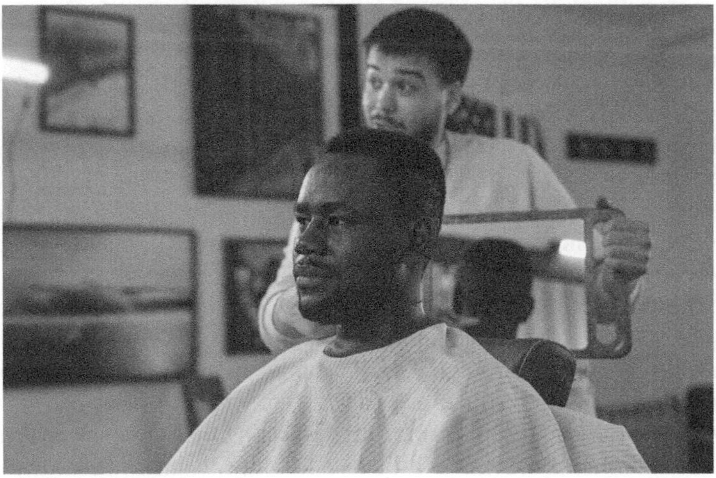

Figure 2.7 Inside a Black barbershop. Photo from Shutterstock.

Los Angeles area. Consistent with larger demographic data demonstrating that African American males are disproportionately affected by higher rates of uncontrolled hypertension, all participants enrolled in the study had a baseline systolic blood pressure of 140 mm Hg or higher. For the study's intervention, researchers enlisted the help of trusted barbers within the community to encourage patrons to meet with pharmacists stationed within these barbershops. The pharmacists worked in collaboration with primary care providers to monitor blood pressure levels and to prescribe medication. At the end of a six-month period, the mean systolic blood pressure for the intervention group fell an average of 27.0 mm Hg for the intervention group compared to 9.3 mm Hg for the controlled group. What these figures signaled to the researchers was that embedding health interventions in trusted community spaces could serve as a powerful tool for promoting patient health. This tool furthermore lies within specific cultures and communities, once more allowing providers with work *within* culture rather than around it.

As Case 4 illustrates, though, practicing culturally competent communication in the clinic involves more than just knowing what resources can facilitate patient adherence. It also involves a comprehensive understanding of the culturally specific reasons behind a lack of adherence in the first place.

Case 4

Scenario: Mr. Davis is seeing his primary care provider (PCP), Dr. Samuelsen, at an outpatient clinic located in rural Georgia in the U.S. South.

Patient: Mr. Davis is a 72-year-old Black male. He has multiple medical problems, including COPD, for which he uses long-acting bronchodilators daily.

He has a rescue inhaler. He was hospitalized in February for a COPD exacerbation after getting a cold from his grandchildren.

Provider: Dr. Samuelsen is a family practice provider at a faith-based primary care practice. He has been seeing Mr. Davis for about four years since joining the practice from his residency program.

Flu cases are on the rise throughout the region, and this year's strains are particularly virulent. Mr. Davis has chronic obstructive pulmonary disease, and so is already at risk of a severe outcome. His PCP is therefore encouraging him to get the flu vaccine. Mr. Davis continues to decline the vaccine, however, saying he "doesn't trust what's in it." Dr. Samuelsen enumerates the benefits of the vaccine, which far outweigh the risks, but to no avail. Dr. Samuelsen leaves the interaction feeling frustrated and unsure as to what else he can do to promote Mr. Davis' health while at the same time respecting his autonomy as a patient.

Patient autonomy refers to a patient's ability to make their own healthcare decisions in a way that is free from coercion, manipulation, or in some instances, provider persuasion. Dr. Samuelsen ultimately respects Mr. Davis' autonomy—his decision to decline the vaccine—despite the fact that it would greatly benefit him. Yet, Dr. Samuelsen's frustration in the above episode is palpable, and likely comes from the well-intentioned place of simply wanting the best health outcome for his patient. His frustration may soon give way to empathetic understanding, which would, in turn, result in a greater likelihood of patient adherence, if he were to consider the historical interactions of Black men with medicine within the American South. One of the most egregious violations of the trust instilled in the medical institution was the Tuskegee Syphilis Study. The study, originally titled "Tuskegee Study of Untreated Syphilis in the Negro Male," was conducted by the U.S. Public Health Service, and recruited 600 Black men participation in Tuskegee, Alabama (Figure 2.8). Of these 600, 399 were infected with syphilis and 201 were not. Those recruited were done so under the pretense that they were being treated for "bad blood," meaning that they were never informed of their syphilis diagnosis. However, information was not the only thing that was withheld from participants in the study. When a cure in the form of penicillin became available in 1947, this too was withheld from participants so that researchers could observe the effects of the disease upon the body as it progressed. Eventually, the operation was exposed by an epidemiologist, Peter Buxton, which resulted in the forced conclusion of the study, and later, prompted an official apology by then-U.S. president Bill Clinton (Jones, 1993).

While the study resulted in some good in that it led to the formation of institutional review boards (refer to Chapter 1), the toll of Tuskegee was nonetheless great. The trauma of the study spanned generations, as did a deep-seated mistrust of medicine among Black-American patient populations. In referring to Case 4, Mr. Davis' reluctance to receive the flu vaccine may be seen as evident of this legacy. Dr. Samuelsen would therefore do well to seek to reassure Mr. Davis

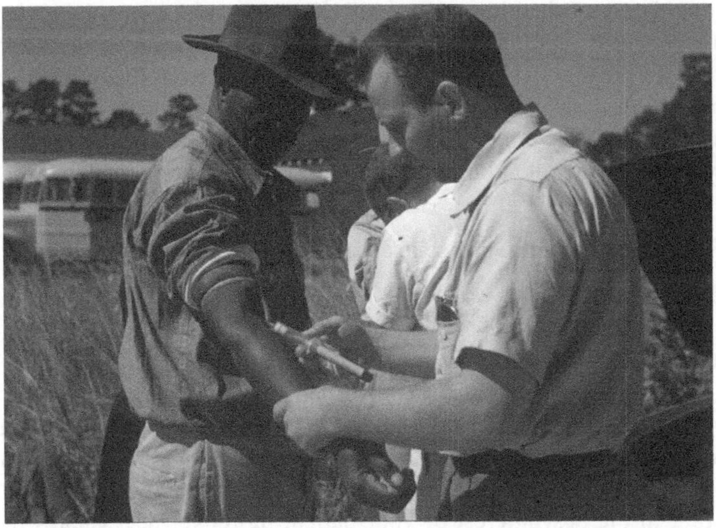

Figure 2.8 A participant in the Tuskegee Syphilis Study gets his blood drawn. Photo from the National Archives.

that he has his best interest at heart. This may look like educating him on the safety of the vaccine, and by detailing the various reviews it must undergo before receiving FDA clearance. Furthermore, in fully appreciating how medicine has historically interacted with certain cultures and communities, Dr. Samuelsen could moreover gently pursue the sources of Mr. Davis' hesitancy with empathy and understanding.

While the Tuskegee experiment represents one of the more high-profile instances of medicine's transgressions, it is far from the first, nor is it likely to be the last. Even prior to Tuskegee, robbing Black graves to supply cadavers for medical education was a rampant practice throughout the U.S. (Washington, 2006). People of color have long had a history of bearing the brunt of medical experimentation for the education and benefit of White patients throughout the world. Take the example of modern-day oral contraceptives. While this medication has been a boon to reproductive autonomy and freedom, its development came at the expense of low-income Puerto Rican women. In 1956, Drs. Gregory Pincus and John Rock chose Puerto Rico as the site for the clinical trial of their new combination estrogen/progesterone pill, largely because "outsourcing" the trials in this way allowed them to circumvent U.S. legal and regulatory frameworks. Hundreds of women were recruited for the trials, most of whom were not properly consented or informed of the risks associated with their participation. And said risks were not insignificant, as these women were given doses near ten times modern-day levels, resulting in extreme side effects (Briggs, 2002).

With the history of the birth control pill trials now told, it may be easier to better understand the complexity behind the Latina woman in clinic, who despite having been pregnant six times, five or which resulted in live births (G6P5), is declining birth control. Certainly, there may be other elements factoring into her decision, which may range from religious beliefs to personal preferences, but the profound impact of cultural legacies must likewise be accounted for.

The Embeddedness of Culture in Healthcare Communication

While these trials were decades ago, the practice of outsourcing clinical trials today is alive and well. In fact, the *New York Times* recently reported on a company that tested its blood-filtering device, which they claimed could cure cancer, in Antigua, out of the reach of U.S. regulators (Carreyrou, 2025). This proves that the exploitation of certain populations for the benefit of others is a perennial issue. Serving as a healthcare provider in today's age therefore means being mindful of these injustices and how they impact the care one receives.

Acting in the best interest of your patient moreover necessitates regarding culture not as something additional to communication in the clinic. Culture is not an "add-on" to the communication process; it is fundamental to it. Culture is not supplemental demographic information; it is the interpretative framework that all health information is filtered through. And acknowledging the immeasurable and varied impact that culture has on one's health is the first step toward providing culturally competent care.

That said, one's cultural identity is just one of the many identities individuals (both providers and patients) bring within them to the clinical setting. Chapter 3 picks up where the present chapter left off by exploring the other identities that enter this space. It addresses how these identities intersect with one another, how they affect the way we see ourselves and how others see us, and more importantly, how we interact with one another from these points of reference.

Glossary

- **Power of attorney**
- **Fiduciary duty**
- **Subculture**
- **Co-culture**
- **Cultural competence**
- **Patient-provider concordance**
- **Machismo**
- **High-context communication**
- **Low-context communication**
- **Acculturation**
- **Ethnocentric**
- **Paternalistic**

- **Cultural relativism**
- **Patient-matched language**
- **Harm reduction**
- **Patient adherence**
- **Patient compliance**
- **Patient autonomy**

Further Reading

- For further information on the UN Declaration of Human Rights, visit: https://www.un.org/en/about-us/universal-declaration-of-human-rights
- For more information on ExThera conducting clinical trials in Antigua, visit: https://www.nytimes.com/2025/01/23/business/exthera-cancer-blood-filtering-device.html
- This chapter touches on longstanding distrust in medicine due to its historical abuses committed against certain groups of people. To learn more about the Puerto Rico birth control trials, visit: https://www.pbs.org/wgbh/americanexperience/features/pill-puerto-rico-pill-trials/

Multimedia Resources

- To learn more about how health, culture, and gender are intertwined, view *Half the Sky*, a documentary about how global gender inequality impacts health outcomes. View an excerpt from the film here: https://www.pbs.org/video/independent-lens-seeking-truth-about-female-genital-cutting-somaliland/
- Another example of how cultural practices and traditions impact health include how members of the Dalit class in India (i.e., "untouchables") are forced to manually clean human waste from latrines as an occupation. Even though the caste system was formally abolished in India decades ago, segregation persists, worsening existing health disparities. To learn more about these health inequities, you can view the short clip featured here: https://www.hrw.org/news/2014/08/25/india-caste-forced-clean-human-waste

Exercise

Classify each of the health beliefs listed below as positive, negative, or neutral. Place a + next to the health belief that should be encouraged to promote patient welfare. Place a – to the health belief that should be discouraged to promote patient welfare. Place a +/– to the health belief that is neutral and does not require intervention.

1 Infants' heads should always be covered.
2 Wearing a red thread around one's wrist will protect against evil.
3 Putting rice cereal in an infant (less than six months old) will help them sleep better.

4 One should never mix meat and dairy in a meal.
5 The best way to get rid of a fever is to heat the body up more—to "sweat it out."
6 Vegetables should be eaten before dairy or meat during a meal.
7 Removing shoes at the door prevents the spread of illness throughout the home.
8 Scraping the skin with a coin or other hard object can release built-up toxins.
9 Women should be confined to the house for the first three months of the postpartum period.
10 Young children should spend as much time as possible outdoors for robust physical health.

Note

1 The capitalization of "Deaf" here was intentional. Many members of this community distinguish between "Deaf" and "deaf," with the former indicating a community defined not by disability, but by their own linguistic system, cultural values, and unique set of practices. The latter, however, encompasses individuals who may have an audiological impairment but do not identify with the Deaf community, proper. For further discussion of the identity politics and terminology of disability, refer to Chapter 3.

References

Airhihenbuwa, C. O. (1990). A conceptual model for culturally appropriate health education programs in developing countries. *International Quarterly of Community Health Education, 11*(1), 53–62.

Alio, A. P., Makhale, L., Hornschuh, S., Hlongwane, K., Otwombe, K., Keefer, M., & Dietrich, J. J. (2019). "Loving the sinner, hating the sin": An investigation of religious leaders' perceived role in the lives of persons living with HIV in Soweto, South Africa. *Journal of Global Health Reports, 3*, e2019021. https://doi.org/10.29392/joghr.3.e2019021

Association of American Medical Colleges. (2023, December 13). *New AAMC data on diversity in medical school enrollment in 2023.* https://www.aamc.org/news/press-releases/new-aamc-data-diversity-medical-school-enrollment-2023

Beauchamp, T. L., & Childress, J. F. (1994). *Principles of biomedical ethics.* Edicoes Loyola.

Bedrosian, S. R., Young, C. E., Smith, L. A., Cox, J. D., Manning, C., Pechta, L., Telfer, J. L., Gaines-McCollom, M., Harben, K., Holmes, W., Lubell, K. M., McQuiston, J. H., Nordlund, K., O'Connor, J., Reynolds, B. S., Schindelar, J. A., Shelley, G., & Daniel, K. L. (2016). Lessons of risk communication and health promotion — West Africa and United States. *Morbidity and Mortality Weekly Report, 65*(Suppl. 3), 68–74. https://www.cdc.gov/mmwr/volumes/65/su/su6503a10.htm

Betancourt, J. R., & Green, A. R. (2010). Commentary: Linking cultural competence training to improved health outcomes: Perspectives from the field. *Academic Medicine, 85*(4), 583–585.

Bigby, J. (Ed.). (2003). *Cross-cultural medicine.* ACP Press.

Briggs, L. (2002). *Reproducing empire: Race, sex, science, and US imperialism in Puerto Rico* (Vol. 11). University of California Press.

British Medical Association. (2024, June 28). British Medical Association. https://www.bma.org.uk/advice-and-support/ethics/medical-students/ethics-toolkit-for-medical-students/cultural-relativism

Carreyrou, J. (2025, January 23). A start-up claimed its device could cure cancer. Then patients began dying. *The New York Times*. https://www.nytimes.com/2025/01/23/business/exthera-cancer-blood-filtering-device.html

Earp, B. D. (2014). *Female genital mutilation (FGM) and male circumcision: Should there be a separate ethical discourse? Practical ethics*. University of Oxford.

Fairhead, J. (2016). Understanding social resistance to the Ebola response in the forest region of the Republic of Guinea: An anthropological perspective. *African Studies Review*, *59*(3), 7–31.

Hadziabdic, E., Albin, B., Heikkilä, K., & Hjelm, K. (2014). Family members' experiences of the use of interpreters in healthcare. *Primary Health Care Research & Development*, *15*(2), 156–169.

Jaeger, F. N., Pellaud, N., Laville, B., & Klauser, P. (2019). Barriers to and solutions for addressing insufficient professional interpreter use in primary healthcare. *BMC Health Services Research*, *19*(753), 1–11.

Jones, J. H. (1993). *Bad blood*. Simon and Schuster.

Kaptchuk, T. J. (1986). The web that has no weaver: Understanding Chinese medicine. *Philosophy East and West*, *36*(1), 67–68.

Kyeong, Y., Yu, M., Tiemeier, H., Bakermans-Kranenburg, M. J., & Setoh, P. (2025). Filial piety across sociocultural context and the life span. *Current Directions in Psychological Science*, *30*(2), 1–8.

National Harm Reduction Coalition. (2024). *Syringe access*. Retrieved May 23, 2025, from https://harmreduction.org/issues/syringe-access/

NHS England. (2025). Workforce Race Equality Standard: 2024 Data Analysis Report for NHS Trusts. https://www.england.nhs.uk/publication/nhs-workforce-race-equality-standard-2024-data-analysis-report-for-nhs-trusts/

Nie, J. B. (2012). The fallacy and dangers of dichotomizing cultural differences: The truth about medical truth telling in China. *AMA Journal of Ethics*, *14*(4), 338–343.

Office for National Statistics. (2022, November 2). *International migration, England and Wales: Census 2021*. https://www.ons.gov.uk/peoplepopulationandcommunity/populationandmigration/internationalmigration/bulletins/internationalmigrationenglandandwales/census2021

Pandya, N. (2023, October 26). Why we shouldn't ask kids to interpret for their parents. *Children's Hospitals Today*. https://www.childrenshospitals.org/news/childrens-hospitals-today/2023/10/why-we-shouldnt-ask-kids-to-interpret-for-their-parents

Pellecchia, U., Crestani, R., Decroo, T., Van den Bergh, R., & Al-Kourdi, Y. (2015). Social consequences of Ebola containment measures in Liberia. *PloS One*, *10*(12), e0143036.

Powell, T. (2006). Cultural context in medical ethics: Lessons from Japan. *Philosophy, Ethics, and Humanities in Medicine*, *1*(4), 1–7. https://doi.org/10.1186/1747-5341-1-4

Reaume, M., Labossière, M. N., Batista, R., Van Haute, S., Tangri, N., Rigatto, C., & Lix, L. M. (2025). Patient-physician language concordance and cardiovascular outcomes among patients with hypertension. *JAMA Network Open*, *8*(2), e2460551.

Saha, S., Komaromy, M., Koepsell, T. D., & Bindman, A. B. (1999). Patient-physician racial concordance and the perceived quality and use of health care. *Archives of Internal Medicine*, *159*(9), 997–1004.

Shell-Duncan, B., & Hernland, Y. (Eds) (2000). *Female "circumcision" in Africa: Culture, controversy, and change*. Lynne Rienner Publishers.

Stanford Geriatric Education Center. (n.d.). *Acculturation*. Stanford University School of Medicine. https://geriatrics.stanford.edu/ethnomed/latino/fund/acculturation.html

Stanford Medicine. (2019). *Impact of cultural factors*. https://geriatrics.stanford.edu/culturemed/overview/introduction/culturalfactors.html

Statistics Canada. (2022, October 26). *Immigrants make up the largest share of the population in over 150 years and continue to shape who we are as Canadians*. https://www12.statcan.gc.ca/census-recensement/2021/rt-td/immigration-eng.cfm

Sundby, J., Essén, B., & Johansen, R. E. B. (2013). Female genital mutilation, cutting, or circumcision. *Obstetrics and Gynecology International, 240421*. https://doi.org/10.1155/2013/240421

Tittley, M. E., Backman, C., Lee, S. H., Gibb, M., & Kehoe MacLeod, K. (2024). Analyzing linguistic and culturally discordant care from the perspectives of nurses and nurse practitioners in Ontario, Canada. *International Journal of Nursing and Health Care Research, 7*, 1547.

U.S. Census Bureau. (2024, April). *The Foreign-Born Population in the United States: 2022* (ACSBR-019). U.S. Department of Commerce. https://www2.census.gov/library/publications/2024/demo/acsbr-019.pdf

U.S. Department of Health and Human Services. (2009). *Federal Policy for the Protection of Human Subjects ('Common Rule')*, 45 CFR 46. https://www.hhs.gov/ohrp/regulations-and-policy/regulations/45-cfr-46/index.html

United Nations. (1948). *Universal Declaration of Human Rights*. https://www.un.org/en/about-us/universal-declaration-of-human-rights

United Nations Population Fund. (2025, February). *Female genital mutilation (FGM): Frequently asked questions*. https://www.unfpa.org/resources/female-genital-mutilation-fgm-frequently-asked-questions

Victor, R. G., Lynch, K., Li, N., Blyler, C., Muhammad, E., Handler, J., & Elashoff, R. M. (2018). A cluster-randomized trial of blood-pressure reduction in black barbershops. *New England Journal of Medicine, 378*(14), 1291–1301.

Washington, H. A. (2006). *Medical apartheid: The dark history of medical experimentation on Black Americans from colonial times to the present*. Doubleday Books.

Williams, N., & Ogden, J. (2004). The impact of matching the patient's vocabulary: A randomized control trial. *Family Practice, 21*(6), 630–635.

World Economic Forum. (2023). *Global Gender Gap Report 2023*. Retrieved from https://www.weforum.org/publications/global-gender-gap-report-2023/

World Health Organization. (2003). Adherence to long-term therapies: Evidence for action. Geneva, Switzerland: World Health Organization. Retrieved from https://apps.who.int/iris/bitstream/handle/10665/42682/9241545992.pdf

World Health Organization. (2023). *Improving maternal health outcomes by addressing female genital mutilation and gender-based violence in Somalia*. In *WHO Results Report 2020 Midterm Review – Country Stories*. Retrieved September 1, 2025, from World Health Organization website.

World Health Organization. (2025, January 31). *Female genital mutilation*. https://www.who.int/news-room/fact-sheets/detail/female-genital-mutilation

World Health Organization. (2025, May 7). *Obesity and overweight*. https://www.who.int/news-room/fact-sheets/detail/obesity-and-overweight

World Medical Association. (2013). *World Medical Association Declaration of Helsinki: Ethical principles for medical research involving human subjects*. https://www.wma.net/policies-post/wma-declaration-of-helsinki-ethical-principles-for-medical-research-involving-human-subjects/

3 Identity in Interaction

Naming, Knowing, and the Language of Clinical Care

Relational Communication

One of the fundamental premises of communication, whether we are talking about health communication or communication in any other context, is that it is relational in nature. The Russian philosopher Mikhail Bakhtin (1986), who is now highly regarded as an early pioneer within the field, once said,

> Every utterance must be regarded primarily as a response to preceding utterances of the given sphere…it is addressed, as if in anticipation, to a response, an answer, a rejoinder… It is oriented toward the anticipated answer-word of the other
>
> (p. 91)

Bakhtin's quote touches on one of the core tenets of communication: that all meaning is relational. Anything one says is always formulated with another individual—real or imagined—in mind. As he puts it, the statement is "is addressed, as if in anticipation, to a response, an answer, a rejoinder." How I anticipate someone might respond to what I say, however, is contingent upon how I see them and how I see myself. Therefore, communication and meaning making are deeply rooted in discussions of identity. Yet, given how scholars understand the concept, it may be more appropriate to term it *identities*.

As the pluralization of this term suggests, any individual is multiple things to different people all at once. The identity they choose to enact at any particular moment in time is dictated by the individual with whom they are in conversation. In the clinic, you may be enacting the identity of a third-year medical student, but at home you are a roommate or significant other. At work, I [Shelby] enact the role of a professor when in the presence of my students, but in my spare time, I primarily assume the identity of a parent. The point is that, at any given time, an individual is multiple things at once. This chapter is concerned with how the various social positions one inhabits influence communication within healthcare settings, and how they moreover intersect with one another so

DOI: 10.4324/9781003654308-3

that this influence often occurs in profound and unexpected ways. The interactions among these different points of reference for being in the world is termed **intersectionality** within the social sciences and humanities. Intersectionality traditionally refers to how individuals can face discrimination and oppression that stem from a combination of multiple identities as opposed to just one alone (Crenshaw, 1991). Applications of the term have since been expanded to simply denote how we are perceived by others and perceive ourselves from multiple perspectives and along myriad lines.

Case 1 illustrates the concept of intersectionality in action with the introduction of Dr. Price, a young orthopedic surgeon and woman of color. It considers how biases along the gendered and racial lines influence notions of professional belongingness. This case is then followed by Case 2, which examines how language choices in the clinic intersect with patient identity so as to validate or disconfirm them. It reviews key terminology for the inclusive practice of medicine and discusses the role that language plays in one's enactment of various identities. Finally, Case 3 introduces a patient with a disability to explore the merits of person-first language and how such language comes up against prevailing societal and medical representations of disability.

Case 1

Scenario: Mr. James Rafferty is a 76-year-old White male admitted to the hospital with abdominal pain caused by diverticulitis. He is lying in a hospital bed and is being seen by Dr. Donnele Price.

Patient: Mr. James Rafferty has hypertension, well-controlled type 2 diabetes (A1c 6.5%), hyperlipidemia, venous insufficiency, and peripheral artery disease with a history of a right lower extremity bypass. This is his third admission for diverticulitis in the past year. He previously had been seen at the local academic hospital, but is admitted to the regional, non-academic hospital.

Providers: Dr. Price is Mr. Rafferty's attending general surgeon and woman of color in her late thirties. She completed a minimally invasive surgery fellowship after her general surgery residency and is a regional expert in robot-assisted abdominal surgery (Figure 3.1).

After an initial history and physical, Mr. Rafferty says he wants to wait to discuss surgery with the "head doctor." Dr. Price calmly states that he is not at a teaching hospital and that she is the only, and "head," general surgeon. She then describes both open and minimally invasive surgical options, including their relative risks and advantages. She offers Mr. Rafferty the opportunity to ask questions. During the subsequent conversation, Mr. Rafferty repeatedly calls Dr. Price "honey," "sweetie," and finally "girl," despite her references to herself as his "doctor."

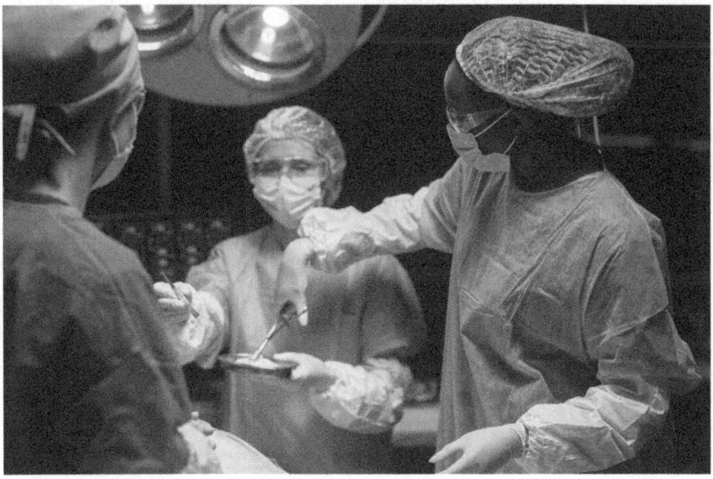

Figure 3.1 A Black female surgeon performing a procedure. Photo from Shutterstock.

In the face of outright misogynistic, derogatory, or otherwise prejudicial language, such as that used by Mr. Rafferty, one may wonder about if the provider in this scenario is compelled—legally, professionally, or ethically—to provide care to the patient, despite such insults and other harmful remarks. Moreover, what is the likelihood that amidst such a backdrop the provider could remain impartial and objective so as to provide patients like Mr. Rafferty with quality care, in spite of their multiple offenses? As will be discussed further in Chapter 7 on communication at the end of life, just as medicine endeavors to uphold patient autonomy, it does the same for providers as well. Providers reserve the right to refuse care (often on moral, ethical, or religious grounds, but some personal as well), yet currently professional recommendations urge these providers to refer the patients for whom they have declined care to a colleague so that they can maintain continuity of care (American Medical Association, n.d.). This is done not only with the individual patient's health and well-being in mind, but to avoid **systemic abandonment**, where certain patient populations are left vulnerable because they cannot reasonably access care, thus worsening many existing health disparities.

While Dr. Price would certainly be within her rights as a clinician to refuse to continue to provide care to Mr. Rafferty, instead of transferring him to the service of a colleague, for the purposes of the present discussion, it is helpful to understand the crux of the problem as lying in a disconnect between Dr. Price's **ascribed** and **avowed identities**. One's ascribed identities are those that the outside world gives to them, and are therefore also labels that the individual themselves have little control over. Examples include "woman," "Asian American," "elderly person," and "person with a disability," to name a few.

In contrast to these ascribed identities are one's avowed identities, which refer to how you see yourself (Martin & Nakayama, 2010). Often, one's ascribed identities and avowed identities do not align, which, in turn, leads to the communication breakdowns and interactional trouble Dr. Price encounters above. While Dr. Price's avowed identity may be that of a competent and skilled surgeon, the identity ascribed to her by some patients, Mr. Rafferty included, is simply as a young Black woman, which they furthermore regard as at odds with her avowed identity.

Dr. Price's story is, unfortunately, a common one. One study published in the *Journal of General Internal Medicine* sought to identify the impact of professional misidentification among resident physicians. The researchers found that 100% of the female residents interviewed reported being misidentified within the last month (usually as nurses rather than physicians), whereas only 49% of their male counterparts encountered the same (Berwick et al., 2021).

In addition to gender, the provider's race or ethnicity also plays a key part in their misidentification by patients. A 2017 report by the Greenlining Institute surveyed 20 female physicians of color to investigate how they understood their professional identity, and how it was understood by those around them. Consistent with Berwick et al.'s (2021) findings, Galace and Calimlim (2017) found that many of the participants reported being mistaken for nurses, administrative staff, and medical students, even after introducing themselves as physicians. They were also met with marked skepticism by both patients and colleagues, who questioned the legitimacy of their diagnoses and treatment plans, and some even went so far as to solicit a second opinion from a White or male provider.

The findings of this report have several important implications, all of which are directly relevant to the case at hand. First, patients may forgo receiving the highest quality care simply because they harbor biases and misconceptions about the competency of the individual providing it. While Dr. Price may be the provider who is most qualified to perform Mr. Rafferty's surgery, Mr. Rafferty's preexisting beliefs may prevent him from receiving such care. Second, given that the study by Galace and Calimlim (2017) noted that colleagues are more likely to question professional assessments and recommendations when they come from individuals from certain social backgrounds, this may present an imminent danger to patient welfare. Such questioning can lead to delays in treatment and prevent the timely provision of services, both of which pose significant concerns for patient health outcomes. More than that, though, when both patients and fellow providers question one's abilities in this way, it may exert a negative impact on the demographic composition of the field as a whole. To illustrate, let us consider the notion of the "Looking Glass Self (Figure 3.2)."

The American sociologist Charles Cooley conceived of the relationship between one's ascribed identity and their avowed identity in terms of the

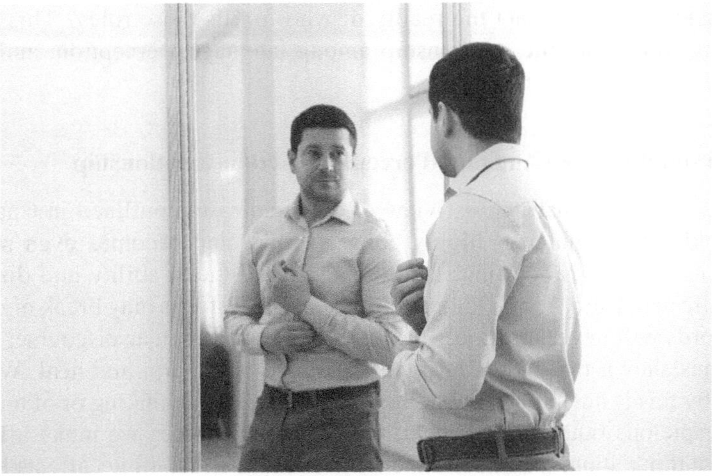

Figure 3.2 A man looks at himself in the mirror. Photo from Shutterstock.

"Looking Glass Self." Cooley (1902) used the analogy of a mirror (i.e., a looking glass) to illustrate how our perceptions of self are influenced by those around us. Much like Bakhtin's statement that all communication is made in response to another anticipated person, Cooley claims that we imagine how we appear to others and then internalize those perceptions into our core conceptions of self. If we are routinely receiving feedback from others that we do not belong, we may be prone to formulate opinions of ourselves that are consistent with the messages we receive. In the case of Dr. Price, if interactions like those that took place with Mr. Rafferty become commonplace, she may eventually come to question her place in the field, or at least her position at her current employer. Prospective providers who share similar social identities may likewise be dissuaded from entering this space, believing them to be inhospitable to providers of a certain gender, racial or ethnic background, and so on. This too has a direct bearing on patient health. As the previous chapter detailed at length, patient-provider concordance figures heavily into intercultural communication in the clinic, which, in turn, exerts a significant impact on patient health outcomes. It stands to reason that if the representation of providers from various backgrounds drastically shifts, these aspects of healthcare will suffer as a result.

When thinking about the sources of the biases embedded in different ascribed identities, several culprits come to mind, from the media to large-scale cultural narratives, to reputations about who belongs in certain specialties (see Bland et al., 1995). But what about the language we use in our everyday interactions? How does the way we communicate about different professional roles impact the reality of who fulfills those roles? This section sets out to explore the relationship among language, perception, and action within healthcare settings.

Understanding the Language-Perception-Action Relationship

In line with the constructivist view of communication outlined in Chapter 1, we hold that language is highly consequential, and becomes even more so when used to talk about matters of health and illness, ability and disability, even life and death. While idioms like "Sticks and stones may break my bones, but words will never hurt me" may circulate in the popular discourse, experience has shown that words have the power to both harm and heal. What we mean by this is not suggestive of the power of positive thinking or of manifesting auspicious outcomes. Instead, the linguistic choices we make affect the way we think about things, and the way we think about things affects how we act with respect to them.

The notion that wording alone can deeply influence how something is regarded—whether than be an individual, a disease, or a healthcare system—is apparent in one of the greatest marketing schemes in history (see O'Connor, 2020). In 1977, a U.S. fish importer named Lee Lantz saw the potential for a widely abundant species of fish to be re-branded into a delicacy and commercial success. The problem, however, lay in its name: Patagonian toothfish. This name did not conjure up associations of gourmet cuisine. So, Lantz renamed the fish "Chilean sea bass," which now graces the tables of fine restaurants across the world. As the case of the Patagonian toothfish shows, a simple linguistic rephrasing can yield remarkable results.

So what might such semantic restructuring look like within the world of medicine? Consider a hypothetical example wherein representatives at the WHO or other comparable organization are deciding how to allocate funds to spur healthcare infrastructure. Officials are deciding between various countries in need of such funds. Some of these countries have been labeled using the now-defunct terminology of "Third World country." Others, however, are classified as "developing nations," and still others are described simply as "under-resourced areas." The different linguistic labels applied to each may result in different tangible outcomes. When compared to "Third World country," "developing nation" may lead one to believe that this option represents a good investment since this country and/or people are working toward progress, whereas the former option is "stuck in its ways." "Under-resourced area" is also likely to yield a favorable result for this particular nation or region, as the wording seems to convey that it just needs material assistance (as opposed to interventions at the structural or political level).

These differences in languaging may exert similar effects across contexts. The same could be said about a provider considering volunteering with relief organizations like Médecins Sans Frontières (Doctors Without Borders). As one could imagine, referring to a region as a "conflict area" as opposed to a "war zone" is much more likely to result in increased recruitment of medical personnel. In the context of disease, specifically, Susan Sontag's (1978/1989) *Illness as Metaphor* and *AIDS and Its Metaphors* problematized popular metaphors for describing diseases like cancer, tuberculosis, and HIV/AIDS, such as the militaristic metaphor that is so often employed. The problem with conceptualizing these diseases as necessitating a "battle" where the body must mount "its defenses" to "attack" the virus or malignant cells is that, as with any war, there are winners and losers. Sontag pointed out that linguistically framing illness in such a way placed the onus on the individual in the "war" against their disease. Should they succumb to this disease, and in extending the metaphor, one could argue that they just did not "fight" hard enough.

As these examples demonstrate, the words we use—in the clinic and everyday life—matter. They can even go so far as to fundamentally shape life trajectories. Let us return to earlier discussions of which career paths may appear open to which individuals. Certain professional trajectories appear accessible to certain people, in large part because of how they are linguistically framed. Within medicine, as with other vocations, the wording used to refer to different roles creates a prototype—a representative example—of the kind of person who assumes that role. **Gender qualifiers** like "*female* surgeon" and "*male* nurse" are commonly used to signal this is an exception to the rule and thus reinforce stereotypes regarding gendered professions within healthcare. In this example, the rule is that surgeons are presumably male and nurses are generally female. These reflections are supported by the academic research on the topic, as one study of AI-generated medical narratives found that the large language models (LLMs) in question used female pronouns (she/her) to refer to nurses 98% of the time, though the use of these same pronouns to refer to doctors ranged from 50% to 84%, and even less so for surgeons (36–80%) (Menz et al., 2024). While this study's findings stem from AI-generated narratives, derived from over 6,000 prompts, since the machine learns from input it can access through all corners of the internet, it is reasonable to conclude that the AI output is consistent with larger societal narratives about different occupations within medicine.

Within my own professional practice, I [Shelby] have witnessed firsthand the far-reaching effects of the biases brought on by simple word choice. For the past 15 years, within my undergraduate and graduate classrooms, I have asked my students to participate in a variation of the Draw-a-Scientist activity. Originally developed by David Chambers (1983), the Draw-a-Scientist program sought to unearth biases embedded in various professional identities by asking students to draw a scientist. Invariably, Chambers found that the scientist was depicted in a stereotypical fashion: as an older White male. In my own applications of this program, I have routinely asked my students to draw a physician and a nurse,

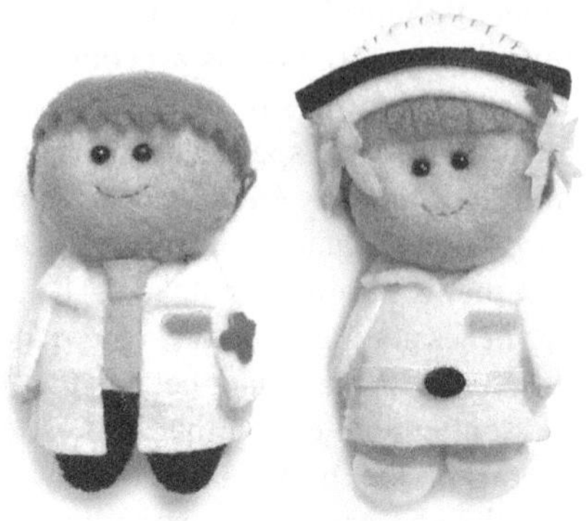

Figure 3.3 A depiction of a doctor and nurse consistent with gender stereotypes.

and in later years, added other occupations like "physician assistant," "ultrasound technician," and so on. Across the many years of using this exercise in the classroom, the gendered trends of certain professions being "male" or "female" have prevailed (see Figure 3.3). That said, in the past few years, the clear demarcation between male-only or female-only occupations has destabilized, perhaps due to the shift toward more inclusive and equitable language within medicine.

Part of making language choices that work toward gender equity in medicine involves avoiding the **gender diminutive**. Mr. Rafferty invokes the gender diminutive when he refers to Dr. Price in infantilizing terms like "sweetie," "honey," and "girl." While on the surface many of these terms may seem like forms of endearment, they can actually work to undermine the status or professional identity of the individual to whom they are directed. The use of gender diminutives toward women in the workplace is common, with women being more often referred to as a "girl" while adult men are rarely referred to as "boys" (Lakoff, 1975). As an important aside, there are regional and cultural variations to consider here. For example, in the American South, terms of endearment like "darling," "sweetie," and "sugar" are not at all unusual (Brown & Levinson, 1987). Whether these terms constitute an instance of patronizing communication, a move toward rapport-building (see Chapter 4), or a **microaggression,** depends entirely on the context.

Microaggressions refer to "daily commonplace, subtle behaviors and attitudes toward others that arise from conscious or unconscious bias" (Ehie et al., 2021). In Case 1, given the overarching context of this communication event and the tenor of the conversation, Mr. Rafferty's use of gender diminutives, coupled with his request to see "a real doctor," may be seen as microaggressions designed to undermine the legitimacy of Dr. Price's professional identity. But within any interaction, there are various communicative resources one can deploy to achieve their goals. So, what resources are available to Dr. Price? She can, as previously stated, refer Mr. Rafferty to another provider on the grounds that she may no longer be able to treat him objectively, given these microaggressions. Alternatively, she could detail her qualifications to Mr. Rafferty, signaling to him that she is more than competent. Finally, she may ask information-seeking questions to determine the root cause of Mr. Raffery's animosity toward her. These insults may stem from latent fears he harbors regarding his impending surgery, and the better able Dr. Price is to identify those fears, the better able she is to allay them.

Communication as a Vehicle for Identity-Affirming Care

In recent years, increasing attention has been devoted to examining microaggressions in healthcare, specifically to inquiring into the linguistic choices providers use to refer to transgender patients. While entirely hypothetical in nature, Case 2 is informed by actual clinical encounters that have been reported to us and illustrates the profound impact that language can have on one's health.

Case 2

Scenario: Mr. Holmes, a transgender male, is seeing Dr. Ari Martinez at an outpatient gynecology practice (Figure 3.4).

Patient: Mr. Holmes, a transgender male, born female at birth, is 39-years-old. He has a history of hypothyroidism on levothyroxine 50 mcg daily. In the past two years, Mr. Holmes has undergone chest masculinization surgery to

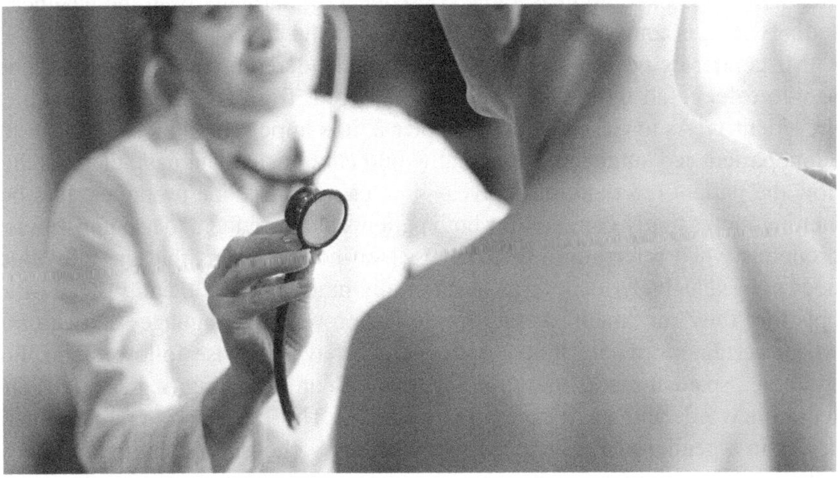

Figure 3.4 A transgender patient undergoing an exam.

remove his breasts and is currently receiving testosterone cypionate 200 mg IM every two weeks.

Providers: Dr. Martinez is an OBGYN practicing in a private outpatient clinic. She is accompanied by Nurse Kelly.

After knocking to see if the patient is covered in his exam gown and drape, Dr. Martinez enters the room with a nurse, and greets the patient by saying, "Hello, Michelle. I'm Dr. Martinez. I see you're here for your annual exam."

The patient quickly interjects, "Actually, it's Michael. I believe that's noted in my chart."

Dr. Martinez says, "Ah, yes, I see. I apologize. Generally, I will start with a breast exam, and then I will perform a pelvic exam."

The patient, Mr. Holmes, responds, "That's fine, but would you mind referring to the area as my 'chest'?"

To this, Dr. Martinzes says, "Yes, of course." She then turns to Nurse Kelly and asks to "prepare a Pap test kit for her."

This exchange portrays Dr. Martinez as rather responsive to the patient's requests for using certain language. For instance, when Dr. Martinez **deadnames** the patient (i.e., she uses the name the patient was assigned at birth and no longer identifies as), the patient indicates her preferred name, and Dr. Martinez responds positively. And again, when the patient requests that Dr. Martinez refrain from using gendered language to describe her chest, given that she has undergone top surgery, Dr. Martinez is equally amiable. However, toward the end of the exchange, we see Dr. Martinez speaking to Nurse Kelly, where she refers to the patient using female pronouns. Given Dr. Martinez's agreeableness throughout the interaction, it is unlikely that this was done with malintent. Yet, as has been demonstrated thus far, words have immeasurable consequences, particularly in the healthcare setting. So, it is concerning that she **misgenders** the patient in this way.

Misgendering occurs when someone uses gendered pronouns (he, him, she, her) to refer to an individual which are different from the gender with which they identify. As in Case 3 within Chapter 2, it is important in these instances to adopt patient-led language. Here, that would entail using language that matches how the patient refers to themselves—i.e., using masculine pronouns. It is becoming increasingly common for both patients and providers to use **non-binary** pronouns when referring to themselves. Non-binary means that the individual does not exclusively identify as traditionally male or female, and instead often opts for "they" or "them" as their preferred pronouns. Languages and cultures where certain words are inherently gendered have likewise followed suit. For example, Spanish marks masculine words with an -o ending (e.g., Latino) and feminine words with an -a ending (e.g., Latina). Those wishing to refer to themselves in a gender-neutral manner, however, may choose to identify as LatinX, with the "X" denoting a shift away from the gender binary implicit in the structure and form of the Spanish language.

Other terms that clinicians are likely to encounter in their practice include various acronyms like, **FTM** and **MTF**, as well as **AFAB** and **AMAB**. FTM stands for female-to-male, indicating that a patient has transitioned, or is currently transitioning from female to male. MTF, however, signals that the patient is currently transitioning or has previously transitioned from male to female. Yet, from a medical standpoint, if the patient possesses organs and anatomical features that are relevant to the care one provides, it would still be essential to know this information. For example, it would be essential to providing sound gynecological care to know that even though Mr. Holmes has removed his breasts and is taking testosterone, he still has a uterus and ovaries, the presence which would necessitate a physical exam. The way that this may be noted in his chart is by referring to Mr. Holmes as AFAB. AFAB stands for "assigned female at birth", and could prompt the provider to inquire about which therapies or surgical interventions the patient has undergone, thus effectively informing their care. In this way, the patient chart[1] can be a powerful and important tool for providing **gender-affirming** care, which the WHO defines as healthcare that "can include any single or combination of a number of social, psychological, behavioural or medical (including hormonal treatment or surgery) interventions designed to support and affirm an individual's gender identity." And while it can be easy to write off these seemingly insignificant linguistic choices as inconsequential, as Loder (2019) writing for the *British Medical Journal* notes, "The pronouns we use betray our biases." But perhaps more importantly, she continues, "They also shape our view of the world and what is possible." In this way, Loder's commentary calls back to previous discussions of who belongs within medicine and in what capacity.

In this discussion of pronoun use, however, it is important to note even if the patient is **cisgender**, meaning that they identify with the gender that corresponds to their sex at birth, they may still prefer non-binary pronouns. In addition to following patient-led language choices, it is always a good practice to explicitly inquire about patient preferences when in doubt. In the context of Dr. Martinez's interaction with Mr. Holmes, this might look something like, "I see that your chart identifies you as 'Michelle,' but you have introduced yourself here as 'Michael.' Would you like me to make a note of this for you? Also, what pronouns would you prefer I use with you?"

Identity as a Performance Mediated by Communication

This distinction between sex and gender introduces an important avenue for further discussion, given the current chapter's focus on the intersections of identity and communication in the clinic. Most contemporary social theorists hold that identity is something one *does* rather than something one is. What does that mean? Well, if we think back to the discussions at the beginning of this chapter regarding identity as something one enacts in specific settings in the presence of specific others, this take on identity as a performance remains consistent. The difference between sex and gender may be thought of along these lines. **Gender** is part of one's identity that they perform in their daily interactions by way of the clothes they wear, the way they style their hair, even the pronouns they choose to adopt. **Sex**, by contrast, refers to anatomical features, reproductive organs, and hormones.

The American feminist and philosopher Judith Butler is perhaps one of the most well-known pioneers in gender and sexuality studies, and her work, *Gender Trouble*, was instrumental in advancing the notion that one's gender identity is something one performs. In the book, she writes, "Gender is not something that one is, it is something one does, an act… a doing rather than a being" (Butler, 1990, p. 25). The trouble is that in calling it "an act," some have mistakenly interpreted this as meaning that this identity is fake or otherwise a facade that one puts on for others. Butler's intent, however, was to denaturalize gender as we know it. There is nothing, for example, about being born a woman that dictates I must present myself in a feminine way: by wearing makeup, having long hair, and donning dresses. The identity one performs is very much real. But the point here is that my gender identity is something I *choose* to perform—to communicate—through a variety of means through everyday microinteractions.

Sometimes, however, one's gender identity and their sex do not align, as in the case of Mr. Holmes. The International Classification of Diseases (ICD) designates this "gender incongruence" a condition, a disorder, warranting medical intervention and treatment (WHO, 2019). In thinking back on Chapter 1's discussion of medicalization, one could argue that such diagnostic labeling unnecessarily medicalizes an individual's identity expression. However, proponents of such classifications contend such diagnoses allow patients to receive insurance authorizations that grant them the gender-affirming care they desire. Additionally, diagnoses like "gender incongruence" are more favorable in their framing of the condition than its predecessors in the *Diagnostic and Statistical Manual of Mental Disorders (DSM-V)*. In the current *DSM-V*, "gender dysphoria" serves as the equivalent to the ICD's "gender incongruence," with the language of the latter denoting an intentional shift away from pathologization. Prior to the adoption of this terminology, however, previous editions of the *DSM* classified the trans experience as a "gender identity disorder." Yet, advocates pushing for revised terminology took issue with labeling this phenomenon a disorder, as it implied a moral judgment. The evolution of the terminology surrounding trans health reflects a growing trend in medicine to remain mindful of the language used within healthcare interactions, especially as they pertain to patient and provider identities alike.

The notion that identity is something one enacts, something they perform, is not just applicable to gender. In many ways, you will be called upon and expected to "act like a doctor/nurse/technician." In her book, *Communicating in the Clinic: Negotiating Front Stage and Backstage Teamwork*, Ellingson (2005) recounts an interaction she observed when researching the communication that happens between medical professionals backstage, out of the view of patients (see Chapter 5 for more on this topic). In this interaction, an attending chastises a resident for expressing uncertainty in front of the patient, instructing the resident to "speak like a doctor." Again, we can see here how communication, identity, and the performance of that identity all intersect. The identity of a doctor is largely socially defined as one that exudes a confident, assured, and knowledgeable communication style. For some, like the attending in this scenario, properly enacting the professional identity of a doctor entails utilizing a communication style such as this. When the resident physician fails to adopt this manner in speaking, and thus fails to properly perform the social identity ascribed to him, the attending attempts to correct this behavior. Within this episode, though, one can see how the expectations attached to certain identities become problematic, and in this case, potentially dangerous. Not feeling secure or able to express doubt or uncertainty may lead the resident physician to speak or act in an overconfident way, which, in turn, can result in misinformed health decisions and poor patient outcomes

The close connection among identity, communication, and health is further illustrated by Case 3. Case 3 features a young patient with a disability and raises the questions of how providers should refer to patients' disabilities in conversation and why this matters.

Case 3

Scenario: Johannes Van Steeden is a 28-year-old male with a history of cerebral palsy. He is accompanied by a friend, Julia. He is being seen at a dermatology office by Dr. Lucy McFadden for a yearly dermatologic exam. Johannes' father has a history of squamous cell carcinoma (Figure 3.5).

Dr. McFadden asks Mr. Van Steeden if he can "hop up to the exam table." He manages to lift himself to the table with some trouble, and Dr. McFadden says, "That's great. You didn't even need my help at all."

Patient: Johannes is a 28-year-old male with cerebral palsy. He has weakness in his left leg and arm with a severe left arm contracture. He occasionally uses a wheelchair and wears an ankle-foot orthotic on his left ankle.

Provider: Dr. McFadden is a dermatologist and has been in her current practice for 12 years.

During the course of the upper body exam, Dr. McFadden tells Johannes that she worked with disabled people as a volunteer before medical school. Johannes very quickly corrects her, saying, "I'm actually a person with a disability." Dr. McFadden quickly apologizes and does the rest of the exam quietly. At the

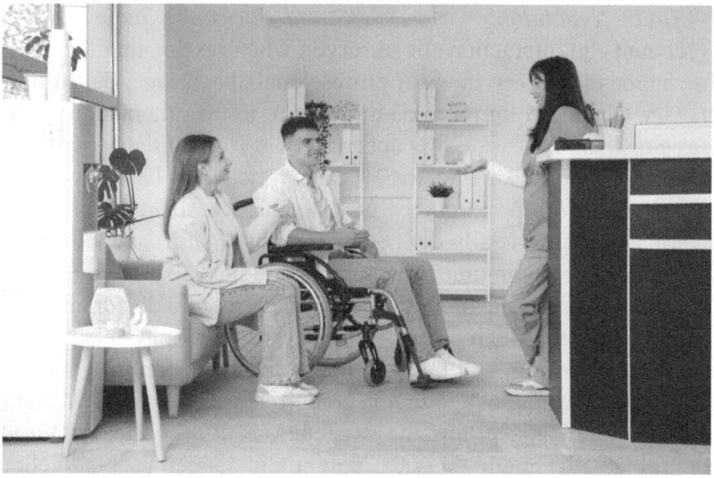

Figure 3.5 A wheelchair user arriving for a health visit.

end, she tells Johannes that he can put his shirt back on. As he does so, she says, "it's really amazing how you've adapted to your arm to get your shirt on so easily."

Unbeknownst to Dr. McFadden, she was entering into a decades-long debate within communities of disability and scholars of disability studies. This debate centers around the language used to refer to people with disabilities, and grounds the discussion of such firmly in issues of identity politics. **Identity politics** refers to "political activity and theorizing founded in the shared experiences of injustice of members of certain social groups" (Heyes, 2024). For many, the injustices shared by different groups are reflected in the language used to refer to their experiences. This is the case with the two camps that prevail within communities of disability—those who prefer "disabled people," and those who endorse "people with disabilities." The first phrasing is widely used throughout the U.K. (but less commonly in the U.S. and Canada), as it was popularized with the advocacy work of Mike Oliver. Oliver, a British disability sociologist, championed this terminology over alternative phrasings because, as he saw it, this wording highlighted how exclusionary systems actively disabled people. The U.K.-based Union of the Physically Impaired Against Segregation (UPIAS) along with Oliver are credited with developing the **social model of disability** that argues that one's impairment (e.g., the inability to walk) only becomes disabling when met with oppressive social structures (e.g., building designs that lack accessible entrances). The cover art for his landmark text, *The Politics of Disablement*, illustrates this distinction between these two concepts (impairment v. disability) by showing a wheelchair

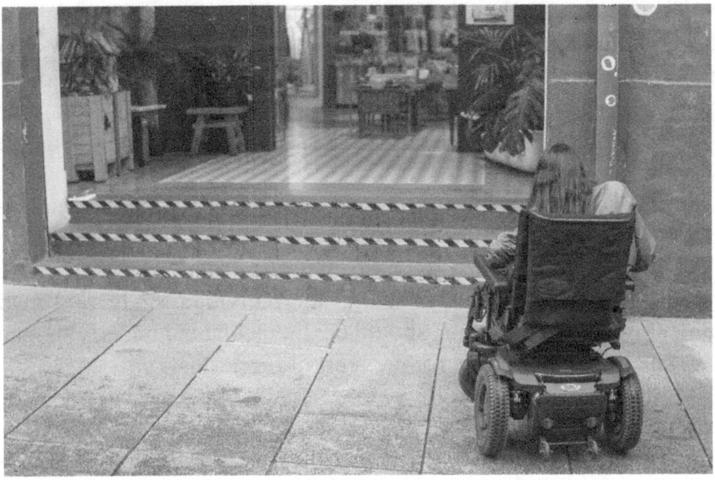

Figure 3.6 A wheelchair user unable to access a store due to stairs. Photo from Shutterstock.

user confronting a flight of stairs (Oliver, 1990) (for a similar example, reference Figure 3.6 above). On its own, the impairment itself is not disabling; yet, when it is met with ableist social systems (here, a flight of stairs), it becomes so.

If you are practicing in the U.S. or Canada, as a result of the different trajectories toward disability advocacy witnessed in these countries and the U.K., patients may prefer **person-first language**. The wording surrounding the use of assistive devices, technologies, and other aids may also be influenced by each country's respective history in the disability rights movement. In the U.S., where it is commonplace to put the person first and the disability second, "wheelchair user" is often more commonly employed in lieu of "person in a wheelchair." With the former, the individual is not defined by their disability, and the assistive device is simply a tool, not something they are confined by/to.

The central role of language in disabled identities may also be observed in the case of "Deaf v. deaf." Within communities of individuals with hearing impairments, "deaf," as denoted by a lowercase "d," refers simply to one's audiological status, which is often defined in medical terms as some form of hearing loss. "Deaf" with a capital "D" signals membership within a particular culture, defined by their own unique language (e.g., sign language) and values. One of these values, in fact, is that members of the Deaf community do not see their hearing loss as a deficit or disability. Rather, for them, it is simply difference. Given the unique set of values often endorsed by the Deaf community, providers should be aware that many medical interventions designed to restore hearing are not always viewed favorably among this population (Ladd, 2003).

Part of the reason for that the Deaf community rejects medical interventions like cochlear implants is because those who subscribe to this view may see it as upholding a **biomedical model of disability**. This paradigm of disability is arguably the most pervasive and certainly the most germane to aspiring and practicing medical providers. Berghs et al. (2016) define this model as seeing

> impairment as a consequence of some 'deviation' from 'normal' body functioning, which has 'undesirable' consequences for the affected individual. Impairment is seen as indicative of an underlying physical abnormality (pathology), located within the individual body, and medical treatment, wherever possible, should be directed at the underlying pathology in an attempt to correct (or prevent) the abnormality
>
> (p. 26)

Many critics of the biomedical model of disability ground their arguments in the anti-medicalization movement discussed in Chapter 1. For them, this representation of disability authorizes medicine to enter into an individual's life in order to treat the disability, and in doing so, effectively broadens its market of prospective patients. Case 3 illustrates the pitfalls of this model from a distinctly medical perspective. In inadvertently reducing the patient to their disability (one might say, designating them a CP patient as opposed to a patient with CP), Dr. McFadden is reaffirming a biomedical model of disability that defines it as an individual problem in need of correction. More than that, however, the narrow view of disability advanced by this model is what leads Dr. McFadden to only focus on the patient's disability, to the exclusion of other significant symptoms, unrelated to it. Unfortunately, this patient's story is all too common and well-represented in the literature, with scholars like Dell'Armo & Tassé (2024) finding evidence of routine "diagnostic overshadowing" of an existing intellectual disability, which causes providers to overlook symptoms attributable to other underlying issues. One can envision the grave consequences of this if these symptoms were to stem from a life-threatening illness or condition. All of this underscores the importance of clinicians reflecting thoughtfully on how disability is represented in both large-scale societal narratives and everyday conversation for patient health.

Yet, the biomedical of disability is but one of many longstanding narratives of disability. One that is even older, yet equally as prevalent within global societies, is a representation of disability as the physical manifestation of a moral failing. As Davis (2013) notes, for much of recorded history, specifically prior to the Enlightenment, disability was frequently seen as an external manifestation of internal sin or moral transgression. In Judeo-Christian traditions, for example, a child born with an impairment was often interpreted as evidence of "sins of the father." Within this context, disability was seen as a proof that the child's parents had transgressed a natural law or the moral order. And while now it is easy to condemn these early attempts at making sense of difference as archaic and ill-informed, the narratives of disability often advanced by modern media do not represent a significant departure.

Captain Hook from Disney's adaptation of *Peter Pan*, Darth Vader of the Star Wars series, most of the James Bond villains, and Scar in the *Lion King*—all of these figures adhere to the common trope of disability as a bodily expression of a supposedly faulty moral compass. Why this matters for the more local level of clinical practice is that these pervasive, large-scale narratives of disability inevitably "trickle down" to everyday interactions. While most medical professionals would ideally demonstrate a certain self-awareness that prevents them from moralizing a patient's disability in this way, there is often another similarly harmful cultural narrative at play: the **supercrip narrative** (Figure 3.7).

Scholars working within disability studies have used the supercrip narrative to describe media portrayals of individuals with disabilities that, on the surface, attempt to be praiseworthy, but in reality, end up being more patronizing than anything else. The supercrip narrative commends people with disabilities for doing things that would otherwise not be noteworthy: driving, socializing, walking, even dating. This narrative forms the premise of recent Netflix shows like *Down with Love* and *Love on the Spectrum*. The first of these series follows individuals with Down Syndrome as they explore romantic relationships. While this show has been positively received by disability advocates for promoting the visibility and representation of people with disabilities within mainstream media and portraying them as romantically inclined when common stereotypes infantilize them or deem them asexual (Kim, 2011), others may find these representations

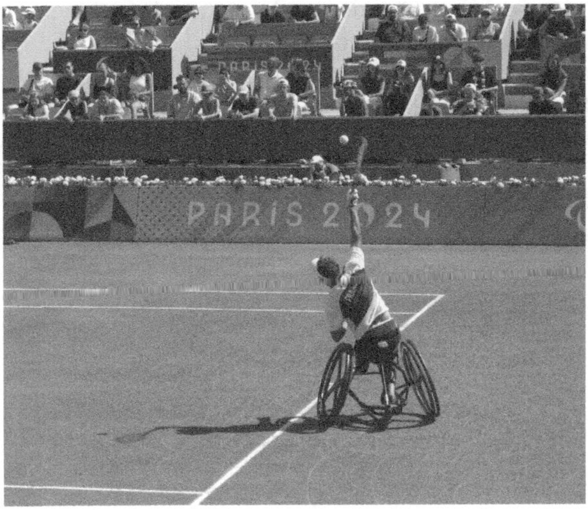

Figure 3.7 A Paralympic athlete playing tennis. Photo from Shutterstock.

problematic. Dating, interacting with others, and even falling in love are not noteworthy actions for a person without a disability, some might argue, so why should they be for people with disabilities?

A similar argument may be made for *Love on the Spectrum*, another Netflix series that features people with autism spectrum disorder (ASD), who are pursuing romantic relationships. Once again, the cast is portrayed as inspirational for doing ordinary things, and thus the show closely adheres to the supercrip narrative. We can see how these larger narratives influence Dr. McFadden's interactions with Mr. Van Steeden in that she likewise inadvertently employs a supercrip narrative when she praises the patient for getting on the exam table without assistance. Although providers certainly want to be encouraging in their interactions with patients, and in specialties like oncology, pain management and rehabilitation, and orthopedics, this is a core part of their ethos, medical professionals should also be mindful of how such praise may be differently interpreted by different populations.

In all of these discussions of disabled identities, terminology, and communicative representations, however, one element has been neglected—the fact that, regardless of critiques of disability framed as a medical problem, people with disabilities still need medical care. In fact, isn't this why Mr. Van Steeden is seeing Dr. McFadden in the first place—because he needs care? This line of reasoning represents one of the greatest shortcomings of the social model's rejection of a biomedical model. That is why, in recent years, disability scholars and advocates have attempted to reconcile the social and biomedical models by acknowledging that, at times, disability has a place within medicine, and though medicine has harmed people with disabilities at several junctures throughout history, it has also done a lot of good, improving the quality of life for countless individuals. Recognizing this, scholars like Martiny (2015) have advanced an embodied or experiential view of impairment that concedes the physical implications of disability that so often require medical assistance, while at the same time remaining cognizant of the pronounced structural barriers that people with disabilities face. This take on disability, rooted in the individual's lived experiences with it, acknowledges that therapies targeted toward ameliorating the symptoms of a disability or improving the individual's quality of life may, at times, necessitate a medicalized view of the impairment. However, it is careful to simultaneously validate alternative representations of disability grounded in the broader social contexts that shape how disability is understood and responded to—both within and beyond the clinic.

The Language of Belonging and Patient Health Outcomes

Talk is cheap. Actions speak louder than words. You can talk the talk, but can you walk the walk? These are just a few of many cultural idioms that belie our assumptions regarding the impact of language and communication. However, as this chapter has set out to do, seemingly insignificant linguistic choices and communication moves within interaction profoundly influence who we believe ourselves and others to be. In tracing the histories of different social groups as they advocate for equal rights, social inclusion, and better health outcomes, however, this chapter has sought to illustrate the central role that communication plays in achieving these goals. In many ways, the language we use in medicine draws boundaries within and around it.

As Case 1 demonstrated, for example, the language used to refer to certain roles within the field and practice intimates gendered assumptions about the profession. The use of gender qualifiers like "female doctor" or "male nurse," though often presented as neutral descriptors, subtly reinforces preconceived notions about who belongs within medicine and in what capacity. Cases 2 and 3, by contrast, illustrated the importance of both patient-matched language for patient-centered care, and for making communicative choices that allow the patient to identify in multiple different ways. Using inclusive language and mirroring patients' preferred terminology have, perhaps not surprisingly, been tied to higher patient satisfaction levels (Beach et al., 2005). While the rapport-building function of this communication in the clinic is admirable in how it instills trust within medicine as a whole (which is especially important for patient populations who have had a troubled history with it), its effects are correlated with markedly improved health outcomes (Stewart, 1995). When a patient is more satisfied with their provider and the care that they receive, they are more likely to feel comfortable raising concerns or divulging private but clinically pertinent information, and to adhere to provider recommendations and treatment plans. Additionally, for vulnerable populations like trans patients and patients with disabilities, both of whom already suffer from higher depression, anxiety, and suicide rates than the general population (Reisner et al., 2016), providing care with a communication-based focus that validates their identity becomes not just an added bonus, but as vital as any medication or other therapy. Thought of in these terms, then, sound linguistic and communicative choices in the clinic are not just a *part* of medicine; they are medicine itself.

Glossary

- **Intersectionality**
- **Systemic abandonment**
- **Ascribed identity**
- **Avowed identity**
- **Gender qualifiers**
- **Gender diminutive**
- **Microaggression**
- **Deadnames**

- **Misgendering**
- **Non-binary**
- **FTM/MTF**
- **AFAB/AMAB**
- **Gender-affirming care**
- **Cisgender**
- **Gender**
- **Sex**
- **Identity politics**
- **Social model of disability**
- **Person-first language**
- **Biomedical model**
- **Supercrip narrative**

Discussion Questions

1. List some of your avowed identities. Now list some of your ascribed identities. Looking at them side by side, consider (a) how they align or conflict with one another, and (b) how they may show up in the clinical space.
2. Outside of the militaristic metaphor that Sontag describes, what are some of the more common metaphors we use to describe various diseases and the state of illness?
3. Metaphors are ideal communicative tools to promote mutual understanding and facilitate patient comprehension. Recognizing the drawbacks of a militaristic metaphor to describe disease effects and progression, what alternative analogies might you use in your clinical practice?
4. Can you think of any other media representations where the character's disability is used as shorthand for villainy? What about instances where one "overcomes" their disability to do unremarkable things? How do you see these narratives potentially impacting communication with patients with disabilities?

Exercise

Take a moment to conduct your own Draw-a-Scientist exercise. Ask those around you to draw various occupations and professional roles within medicine. Do you notice any trends? If so, what are the implications of these trends for both the future healthcare workforce and patient health?

Further Reading

- To learn more about how language affects perception in healthcare, read Susan Sontag's foundational texts *Illness as Metaphor* (1978) and *AIDS and Its Metaphors* (1989).

- For a more in-depth overview of the social and biomedical models of disability, consult this NIH publication by Hogan (2019): https://pmc.ncbi.nlm.nih.gov/articles/PMC6312522/#:~:text=8,9

Multimedia Resources

- View the trailer for the above-referenced Netflix show *Love on the Spectrum* here: https://www.youtube.com/watch?v=uLPRvmpwNHg
- View the trailer for *Down with Love* (Netflix) here: https://www.youtube.com/watch?v=yQg4rshzL-4

Note

1 The chart as an active "participant" in healthcare communication, a mediating agent, and resource for both patients and providers is discussed in greater length in Chapter 6.

References

American Medical Association. (n.d.). *AMA Code of Medical Ethics: Opinion 1.1.7 – Physician exercise of conscience*. https://code-medical-ethics.ama-assn.org/ethics-opinions/physician-exercise-conscience

Bakhtin, M. M. (1986). *Speech genres and other late essays* (V. W. McGee, Trans.; C. Emerson & M. Holquist, Eds.). University of Texas Press. https://doi.org/10.7560/720466

Beach, M. C., Sugarman, J., Johnson, R. L., Arbelaez, J. J., Duggan, P. S., & Cooper, L. A. (2005). Do patients treated with dignity report higher satisfaction, adherence, and receipt of preventive care? *The Annals of Family Medicine*, *3*(4), 331–338.

Berghs, M., Atkin, K., Graham, H., Hatton, C., & Thomas, C. (2016). Implications for public health research of models and theories of disability: A scoping study and evidence synthesis (Public Health Research, No. 4.8). NIHR Journals Library. https://www.ncbi.nlm.nih.gov/books/NBK378951/

Berwick, S., Calev, H., Matthews, A., Mukhopadhyay, A., Poole, B., Talan, J., & Smith, C. C. (2021). Mistaken identity: Frequency and effects of gender-based professional misidentification of resident physicians. *Academic Medicine*, *96*(6), 869–875.

Bland, C. J., Meurer, L. N., & Maldonado, G. (1995). Determinants of primary care specialty choice: A non-statistical meta-analysis of the literature. *Academic Medicine*, *70*(7), 620–641. https://doi.org/10.1097/00001888-199507000-00013

Brown, P., & Levinson, S. C. (1987). *Politeness: Some universals in language usage*. Cambridge University Press.

Butler, J. (1990). *Gender trouble: Feminism and the subversion of identity*. Routledge.

Chambers, D. W. (1983). Stereotypic images of the scientist: The draw-a-scientist test. *Science Education*, *67*(2), 255–265.

Cooley, C. H. (1902). The looking-glass self. *The Production of Reality: Essays and readings on Social Interaction*, *6*(1902), 126–128.

Crenshaw, K. (1991). Mapping the margins: Intersectionality, identity politics, and violence against women of color. *Stanford Law Review*, *43*(6), 1241–1299.

Davis, L. J. (Ed.). (2013). *The disability studies reader* (4th ed.). Routledge.

Dell'Armo, K., & Tassé, M. J. (2024). Diagnostic overshadowing of psychological disorders in people with intellectual disability: A systematic review. *American*

Journal on Intellectual and Developmental Disabilities, 129(2), 116–134. https://doi.org/10.1352/1944-7558-129.2.116

Ehie, O., Muse, I., Hill, L., & Bastien, A. (2021). Professionalism: Microaggression in the healthcare setting. *Current Opinion in Anesthesiology, 34*(2), 131–136.

Ellingson, L. (2005). *Communicating in the clinic: Negotiating frontstage backstage teamwork.* Hampton Press.

Galace, A., & Calimlim, I. (2017). *Breaking down barriers for women physicians of color.* The Greenlining Institute. https://greenlining.org/wp-content/uploads/2017/10/Breaking-Down-Barriers-for-Women-Physicians-of-Color-1.pdf

Heyes, C. (2024). Identity politics. In E. N. Zalta & U. Nodelman (Eds.), *The Stanford encyclopedia of philosophy* (Winter 2024 ed.). Stanford Encyclopedia of Philosophy.

Hogan, A. J. (2019). Social and medical models of disability and mental health: Evolution and renewal. *CMAJ, 191*(1), E16–E18.

Kim, E. (2011). Asexuality in disability narratives. *Sexualities, 14*(4), 479–493.

Ladd, P. (2003). *Understanding deaf culture: In search of deafhood.* Multilingual Matters.

Lakoff, R. (1975). *Language and woman's place.* Harper & Row.

Loder, E. (2019). Time's up for he and him as the default pronouns for doctors. *BMJ, 367.* https://doi.org/10.1136/bmj.l6565

Martin, J. N., & Nakayama, T. K. (2010). *Intercultural communication in contexts.* McGraw-Hill.

Martiny, K. M. (2015). How to develop a phenomenological model of disability. *Medicine, Health Care and Philosophy, 18*(4), 553–565.

Menz, B. D., Kuderer, N. M., Chin-Yee, B., Logan, J. M., Rowland, A., Sorich, M. J., & Hopkins, A. M. (2024). Gender representation of health care professionals in large language model-generated stories. *JAMA Network Open, 7*(9), e2434997.

O'Connor, P. (2020, July 17). Disease branding 101: Marketing medical conditions and the medications to fix them. Psychology Today. https://www.psychologytoday.com/us/blog/philosophy-stirred-not-shaken/202007/disease-branding-101

Oliver, M. (1990). *The politics of disablement: A sociological approach.* St. Martin's Press.

Reisner, S. L., Poteat, T., Keatley, J., Cabral, M., Mothopeng, T., Dunham, E., & Baral, S. D. (2016). Global health burden and needs of transgender populations: A review. *The Lancet, 388*(10042), 412–436.

Sontag, S. (1978). *Illness as metaphor.* Farrar, Straus and Giroux.

Sontag, S. (1989). *AIDS and its metaphors.* Farrar, Straus and Giroux.

Stewart, M. A. (1995). Effective physician-patient communication and health outcomes: A review. *CMAJ: Canadian Medical Association Journal, 152*(9), 1423.

World Health Organization. (2019). *Gender incongruence and transgender health in the ICD* [Frequently asked questions]. World Health Organization. Retrieved June 10, 2025, from https://www.who.int/standards/classifications/frequently-asked-questions/gender-incongruence-and-transgender-health-in-the-icd

4 Disseminating Information and Building Relationships

The Report and Rapport Functions of Communication

Communication Is Constant

The Austrian-American psychologist Paul Watzlawick and colleagues once famously declared, "One cannot not communicate" (Watzlawick et al., 1967). By this, Watzlawick meant to convey several things, the first of which is that even when we think we are not communicating something, we undoubtedly are. Anyone who has been the recipient of the "silent treatment" from a friend or loved one knows that this lack of communication, in fact, communicates the individual's message (whether that be anger, resentment, or frustration) loud and clear. This premise is likewise reflected in some of the cultural idioms introduced in the previous chapter, such as "Actions speak louder than words." Watzlawick's statement about the nature of communication also suggests that communication occurs through several channels, or modes, not all of which are always consistent with one another in terms of the message they impart. In fact, this is how sarcasm works; we are able to discern another person's true meaning by detecting the discrepancy between the content of the message being delivered and its mode of delivery (i.e., the tone and rate of speech, as well as accompanying facial expressions).

Indeed, Watzlawick's statement encourages us to think about the many various channels through which communication can transpire. Often, people think of communication as occurring through oral or written means, as unfolding through conversation or written correspondence. And while this certainly constitutes a bulk of the everyday communication in which we are engaged, so much of what we communicate to others—in the clinic and beyond—occurs through nonverbal means, from the way we style our hair, to the facial expressions we adopt, to the objects (e.g., computers and notepads) that we enlist as "props" to aid in our interaction. Communication scholars have long debated how much of communication is nonverbal, with often-cited but much-contested figures placing estimates at 93% (Burgoon et al., 2021). And while scholars may quibble over the accuracy of this number, they by and large agree that the nonverbal aspects of communication exert a profound effect on processes of

DOI: 10.4324/9781003654308-4

meaning making, which is precisely why this topic figures prominently in the present chapter.

This chapter explores all of the above-described facets of communication by offering an in-depth look at the two functions of communication: the **rapport** function and the **report** function. The report function of communication is likely what comes to mind for most people when they think of the purpose of communication. According to this view, communication is mere message transmission and information dissemination. Listing out the potential side effects of a medication on its labeling or in promotional literature, informing a patient about a potentially upsetting diagnosis, or generating an after-visit summary to include in a patient's electronic health record—all of these examples would qualify as fulfilling the report function of communication.

Rapport, however, refers to the relationship-building aspect of communication. This aspect of communication is less concerned with the raw information conveyed in interaction, but more so with how communication events work in service of bringing individuals together (or pushing them apart, for that matter). Calling or texting your parents or siblings every day is a great example of this type of communication. In such instances, it is usually not what is being said that matters, but the act of routinely reaching out that does. In the clinical setting, mundane pleasantries like small talk about the patient's family, work, or upcoming travel plans may fall into this category. While often not diagnostically relevant, this sort of communication may still hold utilitarian value since as previous chapters have established, patients are much more likely to feel comfortable divulging personal information or adhering to a provider's treatment plan when they feel they have a good relationship with them.

It is important to note that these two levels of communication are always operating in tandem with one another. Therefore, consistent with how the report and rapport functions of communication operate in reality, this chapter discusses both levels of communication simultaneously, in order to better explore how they mutually influence one another. Thus, while Case 1 exemplifies several aspects of the report function of communication, there is inevitably a rapport function of communication at work as well.

These broader discussions of the report and rapport functions of communication are divided up into subsections covering various aspects of the interactive process. The first seeks to provide greater context for understanding these communicative operations by providing a background of popular models for conceptualizing communication itself. After detailing these models' basic premises, outlining salient critiques, and considering how they endure within medicine, we then aim to refine communication, more generally, into the multiple elements that compose it. We begin by exploring chronemics—that is, the temporal elements of communication. Embedded within these reflections of how socially constructed understandings of time impact interpersonal relations within health contexts is an additional acknowledgment of how culture enters in this regard. The following section is reserved for examining the effects of proxemics, kinesics, and tactile communication upon communication in the clinic. This section is therefore largely concerned with how patients and providers negotiate the use of space, attach meaning to facial expressions and gestures, and employ touch toward multiple ends. The chapter then proceeds to consider how artifactual communication—i.e., communication via inanimate objects like attire and exam room design—enables, constrains, or otherwise impacts the nature of communication that unfolds therein. The chapter then concludes with practical takeaways for current and future providers by introducing actionable methods for exploiting both the report and rapport functions of communication in clinical settings.

The Transmission Model of Communication and Its Influence on Medicine

Referring once more to the introductory quote by Watzlawick, this singular statement moreover points to the fact that because not all communication is intentional, our message is not guaranteed to be interpreted in a manner consistent with how we planned. If we assume that "One cannot not communicate," then even when one intends to communicate nothing at all, a message is still being conveyed to one's counterpart, and within the high-stakes context of medicine, it would behoove the provider to reflect on how such a message may be imparted. That said, it is important to note that reflecting upon these processes does not amount to planning or mapping them out. In fact, this misguided belief that a particular communication outcome—whether that be a patient's understanding of the risks associated with a procedure or their adherence to a treatment plan—can be achieved through careful and meticulous communication is pervasive within medicine, and is fundamentally rooted in what Chapter 1 alluded to as the "**transmission model of communication** (see Figure 4.1)."

The transmission model of communication was developed by two telephone company engineers by the name of Claude Shannon and Warren Weaver. In their foundational piece entitled, "A Mathematical Model of Communication," these two researchers posited that communication, in its simplest form, involved a sender who transmitted a message to a receiver (Shannon & Weaver, 1949) Within this model, communication is portrayed as linear and as unidirectional, emanating from the sender to a receiver. Figure 4.1 depicts the transmission model of communication as it is commonly conceived. Within this model, a sender delivers a message to the receiver through a particular channel, such as orally in person, via the patient chart, or through a message sent in an electronic health management portal. To impart the message, the sender (i.e., the provider) must encode the message in a way that is understandable to the receiver; in other words, they must translate the "fuzzy idea" of what they want to communicate into concrete terms—into words. The inverse of this process occurs when the

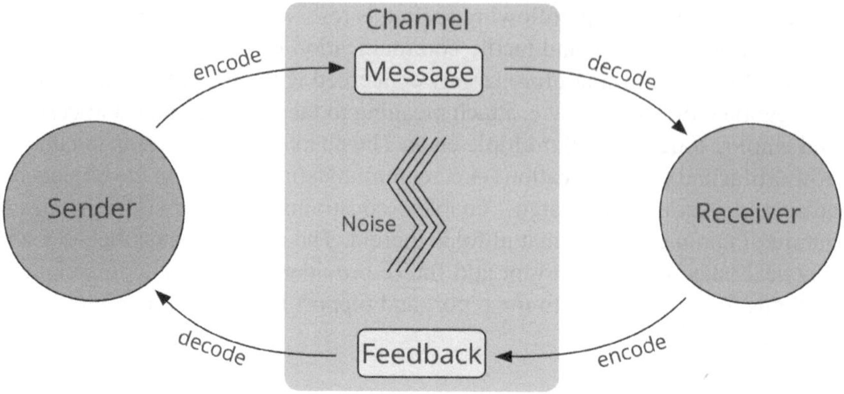

Figure 4.1 The Transmission Model of Communication. Image is author-generated with AI assistance.

recipient of this message receives it and is now tasked with taking those words and decoding, or deconstructing, them in a way that is meaningful to them.

There are, however, several barriers that can interfere with the decoding process. Some may pertain to the process of encoding itself, such as if a provider fails to render information in a way that is accessible to the patient. This often occurs when a provider delivers their message shrouded in medical jargon. This is precisely why several "plain language" initiatives have taken hold throughout Europe (e.g., Germany's National Action Plan for Health Literacy) as well as the U.S. (e.g., plainlanguage.gov).

But there are often other hurdles to understanding that lie outside of the presentation of the message. A common and primary obstacle is what researchers in communication call "noise" (represented in Figure 4.1 as a "lightning bolt"). Communication theorists refine the concept of noise into two distinct subgroups: **psychological noise** and **physiological noise** (Adler et al., 2020). "Physiological noise" refers to external input that may interfere with someone's ability to interpret a message. A rattling air conditioner in the exam room, a person talking in a shared hospital room, or landscape maintenance being performed right outside a clinic are all examples of possible sources of physiological noise. "Psychological noise," however, denotes internal barriers to message comprehension. In a health setting, this may look like a patient who has recently been delivered a poor diagnosis. Perhaps the provider in this scenario continues to elaborate on the prognosis and treatment plan following the diagnosis, but the patient is unable to focus because of the psychological noise brought on by the shock of the diagnosis. Or maybe prior to their appointment, they got into an argument with their significant other, and that is all they can think about at the moment. Or, on the provider's end, perhaps they have been so busy in clinic that they haven't had time to eat today, and therefore, the psychological noise associated with their hunger and thinking about when they will have the opportunity to eat next interferes with their ability to attend to the patient's story. In all of these instances, it is psychological noise that operates as a potential source of interference in the message "transmission."

While this conceptualization of communication may be a helpful starting point, especially for those with little training in communication studies, several scholars have deemed it overly reductive in that it, for one, fails to acknowledge the simultaneous nature of communication. As a message-sender (for our purposes, let's identify this individual as a healthcare provider) is delivering the message, the receiver (here, the patient) is delivering their own. Perhaps they are nodding their head to signal that the provider should continue their explanation of disease etiology. Or maybe they have an expression of confusion written across their face, signaling that they have not fully understood what is being communicated to them. The provider is thus able to recognize and interpret these cues and adjust their message in real time. Maybe this means asking in more overt terms, "Does that make sense?" or altering their word choice so that they adopt everyday parlance instead of medical jargon. Essentially, what we are describing here is the importance of feedback, much of which is often expressed nonverbally, and how senders and receivers offer each other feedback in real time. Feedback not only crucially aids in the report function of communication by ensuring that those involved in the exchange sufficiently comprehend the information presented to them, but it also works in the interest of the relationship-building aspect of the rapport function of communication. Feedback signals attentiveness, a certain degree of responsiveness, and ultimately, mutual respect, and in this way, it can be seen as strengthening the relational foundations upon which clinical communication so vitally depends.

Another primary shortcoming of the transmission model of communication is that it neglects the integral role of human agency. While Chapter 2 briefly alluded to the concept of agency, it did so more or less in passing, and so it is worth unpacking this concept more fully here. **Agency** can be defined as the capacity for an individual to exercise free will over their life and environment. Within medicine, specifically, agency has taken a front-row seat in initiatives and movements like patient centered care and shared-decision-making models. Agency is overlooked in a transmission-based paradigm because such a model assumes that the message recipient will receive the message without further interrogation of it. In other words, this model is predicated on an implicit belief that the patient will agree with, subscribe to, or otherwise resist rejecting the message as it has been conveyed. But common sense tells us that even in the most well-thought-out of interactions, patients—and people in general—often respond to information in unexpected ways, and their questions, signs of disagreement, and outright refusals are all indicators of agency.

Finally, one last critique of this model of communication is that it overlooks the fact that all communication takes place in concrete contexts. Often, these contexts are culturally loaded, as Chapter 2 illustrated, and as Case 1 will demonstrate. The culturally specific nature of communication dictates that certain gestures, actions, and movements are not universally interpreted, and given this, we will once more experience great difficulty in attempting to plan for communication so that it yields a predictable response.

Despite the manifold deficits inherent within this model, however, its presence within medicine and social life at large remains well-defined. In fact, most practitioners in advertising and public relations operate on a transmission model of communication, believing that if we design our ad just so or if we craft our press release as such, we can generate a predictable consumer response—i.e., they will buy our product, elect to receive our service, support our company, and so on. Medicine is likewise not impervious to the follies of the transmission model of communication. Chapter 7 on communication at the end of life, for example, introduces the SPIKES model for Breaking Bad News (Baile et al., 2000). An acronym standing for "setting," "perception," "invitation," "knowledge," "empathy," and "strategy and summary," the SPIKES model was first developed for use in oncological settings as a step-by-step guide advising providers on how to deliver bad news to patients. While the more contextual components of this model, and subsequent renditions like the COMFORT model (Wittenberg et al., 2016), are discussed in greater depth in Chapter 7, our reason for referencing it here is to illustrate medicine's affinity for predictable, linear representations of communication. These prescriptive approaches to communication, wherein a provider follows a series of pre-established steps in communicating with patients, likewise fundamentally neglects the patient's agency. It positions the patient as an idle recipient of information rather than an active participant in meaning making. The use of acronyms also fits with many other mnemonic-based learning strategies common in medical school (PQQRST for history taking, SOAP note format, IPPA for physical exam, etc.).

Fortunately, theories of communication have not stopped at the transmission model. Instead, contemporary scholarship within communication studies has come to endorse a **constitutive model**. As Craig (1999) puts it, this view of communication asserts that communication cannot be reduced to information transmission; rather, it is the means by which members of a particular society create a shared reality. Embedded within this reality are understandings of "truths" (i.e., what it means to be healthy or sick), the norms that guide professional identities and behaviors (i.e., what it means to be a healthcare provider, to be the patient), and even the communicative behaviors available to them. Under this model, the report and rapport functions of communication mutually influence one another. For example, when clinicians deliver a diagnosis or detail the specifics of a treatment plan, they are not simply conveying biomedical facts, but defining the relational context of the care being provided. Presenting information in such a way that it positions patients as welcome collaborators in shared decision-making processes, outsiders naive to the goings-on of medicine, or even as dependent on the clinician's expertise all construct the relationship between provider and patient. And it is this relationship, as it has thus been defined, that then determines how this information is interpreted and understood.

Shifting now from theories of communication to consider how they enter into clinical realities, we now turn to Case 1. Case 1 introduces the patient, Mr. Carvalho, to continue the discussion of how patients and providers might engage in mutual meaning making to create shared realities. It does, however, pose the implicit question of what to do when those realities are not shared. And in calling back to previous chapters on intercultural communication in the clinic, how might we unearth some of the culturally specific assumptions upon which such realities rest? To respond to these questions, and others, we first consider the influence of **chronemics**, or "the study of the concepts and processes of human temporality, or connections with time, as they are bound to human communication interactions" (Littlejohn & Foss, 2009, p. 97).

Chronemics: Time and Culture in Healthcare Communication

Case 1

Scenario: The visit takes place at a clinic in Hamburg, Germany. Mr. Carvalho is seeing his primary care provider, PA Frank Hamm. This is Mr. Carvalho's third visit this year and he unfortunately has already developed a reputation for tardiness. PA Hamm reminds him that his appointment time was 30 minutes ago. Mr. Carvalho says he knows and is sorry, but he was finishing lunch with his wife. He brought a bag of mangoes as an apology and gives them to PA Hamm (Figure 4.2).

Patient: Mr. Carvalho is originally from Brazil. He arrives late and, upon PA Hamm entering the room, is seated in the swivel chair nearest the computer with the mangoes in hand. He told the intake nurse that his concern is about a change in bowel habits. He has been having more constipation since emigrating to Germany a year ago for work.

Provider: PA Hamm has been seeing the provider since he established care. The provider cares about Mr. Carvalho as a patient but is frustrated that he is consistently late as it affects his care of other patients who are on time.

At first glance, there is much in this scene that may indicate that Mr. Carvalho's established relationship with PA Hamm is, in fact, negatively impacting this interaction and subsequently the provider's ability to deliver care. Mr. Carvalho's habitual tardiness, and his lack of punctuality on this day in particular, may signal to some that he has lost sight of the professional nature of this relationship. However, understandings of **monochronic** and **polychronic** temporal

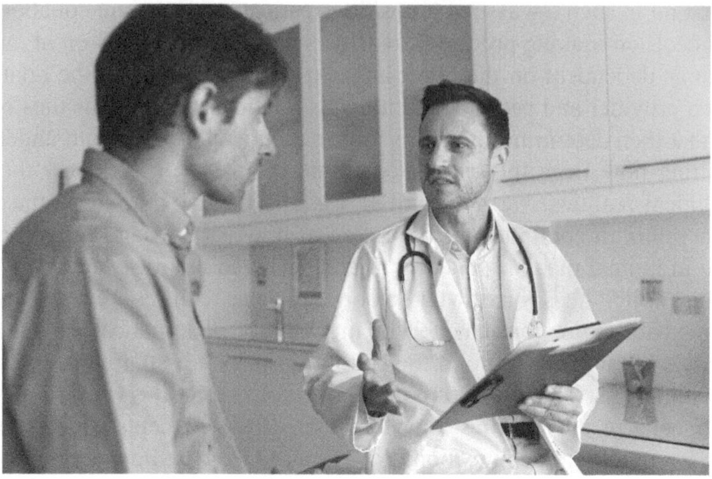

Figure 4.2 Physician interviewing a patient. Photo from Shutterstock.

systems, and how they are reflected in interaction, offer greater insight into the communicative elements at play in this scenario.

Present-day understandings of how culturally informed notions of time may influence human interaction stem from the work of the American anthropologist Edward T. Hall. In his book, *The Silent Language*, Hall (1959) examined how different cultures structure and value time. Hall found that societies characterized by a monochronic understanding of time see it as rigid, highly structured, and generally dictated by clock time. Much of the West, including the U.S., Canada, the U.K., Germany, and Scandinavia, operate on a monochronic temporal system. Much of South and Central America, the Middle East, and India, however, are guided by a polychronic temporal system, where time is viewed in a more fluid manner—a 10:00 am appointment time is thus "10-ish." As Mr. Carvalho is originally from Brazil, where time is typically interpreted along the lines of a polychronic system, his late arrival can be seen as the product of culturally specific understandings of time. The problem, though, lies in what happens when a polychronic perspective meets with a monochronic one. As this clinic is located in Germany, which is, by and large, characterized by a monochronic temporal system, the providers are more likely to regard Mr. Carvalho's behavior as outside of the norm, rude, or downright disrespectful.

In addition to time being more flexible within polychronic societies, it is also seen as secondary to relationships. This may account for why Mr. Carvalho tells PA Hamm that the reason he was late was because he was finishing lunch with his wife. To an individual unfamiliar with the polychronic framework, this may come across as insulting, as if to say that the patient values their other commitments more than the present one. When, however, one comes to understand that relationships are prioritized over time-based obligations within polychronic societies, this presumed blatant disregard for the time of others becomes less offensive.

Proxemics, Kinesics, and Tactile Communication: Space, Movement, and Touch in Clinical Encounters

In addition to popularizing the notion that one's treatment and use of time communicates various messages to others, Hall also advanced the idea that the use of physical space likewise possesses the capacity to communicate via the development of a concept he called **proxemics**. Hall defines "proxemics" as "the interrelated observations and theories of man's use of space as a specialized elaboration of culture." For Hall and modern communication theorists, even those aspects of interaction that one may overlook in communication (to call back to Watzlawick's words introduced at the beginning of this chapter) can express something quite clearly. For instance, Hall was concerned with cultural variations in speakers' use of space, noting that various societies could be differentiated in terms of what he deemed high- or low-contact cultures. Hall observed that people from **high-contact cultures** typically lessened the physical distance between themselves and their conversant, maintained eye contact, and engaged with their interlocutor through touch. Individuals from Mediterranean and Middle Eastern countries often adopt a high-contact communication style, as do individuals from South and Central America (like Mr. Carvalho). Low-contact communication styles stand in contrast to high-contact varieties in that individuals practicing this communication style prefer greater physical distance when interacting, exhibit more restrained facial expressions, and do not engage in handshakes, hugs, or even casual touches as much. The vast majority of North America and Northern Europe would fall into this category of communication, as would many East Asian countries.

One can imagine how these different communication styles may play out in the clinic. In the case where a provider comes from a high-contact culture but is working in a low-contact setting or caring for a patient from such a background, engaging in nonverbal cues and gestures consistent with this culturally specific style may be interpreted as boundary crossing or as a violation of the professional role. Alternatively, if the situation was reversed—in other words, the patient came from a high-contact culture and the provider from a low-contact one—the provider's actions may be interpreted as excessive emotional detachment, marked disinterest, or even downright apathy. Therefore, it is important to account for the cultural dimensions of care, and as the discussion here illustrates, such culturally grounded aspects of communication can fundamentally alter the patient-provider relationship.

Referring once more to Chapter 2, it may be helpful to revisit the concepts of high-context and low-context communication to explore how they align with

Country	Contact	Context	Space (Proxemics)	Movement (Kinesics)	Touch (Tactile)	Clinical Implications
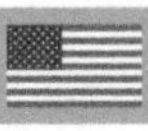	Low	Low	Moderate Distance	Moderately expressive	Minimal	Touch may feel intrusive
	Low	Low	Greater Distance	Reserved	Limited	Positive regard conveyed verbally
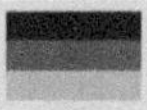	Low	Low	Greater Distance	Precise Gestures	Rare	Direct communication, task-oriented care
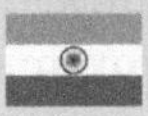	Moderate	High	Variable (often gender-dependent)	Expressive	Context-dependent	Gender, age, and social hierarchy strongly impact interaction
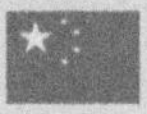	Moderate	High	Variable (urban density)	Controlled	Limited	Indirect communication; patients may avoid direct questioning
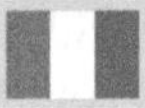	High	High	Low Distance	Highly Animated	Frequent	Warmth and touch expected
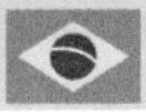	High	High	Low Distance	Expressive	Frequent	Lack of touch may appear overly detached

Figure 4.3 A chart depicting the relationship among culture, touch, and meaning.

high- and *low-contact* communication since the terms share significant overlap (see Figure 4.3 above). As previously noted, Hall first introduced the concepts of high- and low-context communication to examine how meaning is implicitly derived rather than overtly conveyed. Surely, one such way that meaning—for example, the meaning a patient attaches to their relationship to their provider—might be implicitly suggested is through the use of space and nonverbal gestures mentioned above. This brief example also reminds that, much like the quote introduced at the opening of this chapter, meaning is created through multiple channels (e.g., touch and gesture), and such meaning is often more implicit than explicit. Figure 4.3 depicts the relationship among culture, touch, and meaning.

Beyond the cultural dimension influencing how we manage both the physical and psychological spaces between ourselves and others, there is also the matter of interest. When we are interested in someone or something, we engage in what Mehrabian (1971) terms "immediacy" behaviors. These behaviors are meant to signal our interest and often include physically reducing the distance between ourselves and the thing we are interested in. Often, these immediacy behaviors occur below the level of consciousness. You have very likely experienced this phenomenon before. Imagine you are driving and become interested in what the person in the car next to you is doing. What often happens in this scenario is that your car will gradually drift toward that car in the other lane, as we unconsciously close the distance between ourselves and the object of our interest.

So, to move this discussion off the road and into the healthcare setting, specifically, what situations might invite immediacy behaviors? What might they look like? Let's consider if one were to deliver grave news—a serious diagnosis, a high-risk procedure a patient must undergo—the provider may enlist immediacy behaviors to express their vested interest in the topic at hand. As Mehrabian points out, this could look like decreasing the distance between the provider and the patient, perhaps by sitting down, pulling a chair in, and leaning in closer to the patient. Mehrabian notes that another common immediacy behavior involves aligning our head, shoulders, knees, and feet all in the direction of the person or object we are interested in, so providers may consider implementing these nonverbal cues as well.

Artifactual Framing and the Design of Clinical Spaces

But as Case 1 illustrates, it isn't just the two individuals within this health communication episode that are communicating. The room itself is saying something, too. Consider how Mr. Carvalho does not sit where he would normally be expected to—on the exam table, or at the very least, the companion chairs lining the wall of the exam room. Instead, he opts for the swivel stool chair near the computer workstation. Some might see Mr. Carvalho's decision to sit in what otherwise may be designated "the provider's seat" as disrespectful, or as oblivious at best. However, the atypical nature of Mr. Carvalho's use of the clinical space may offer insights into how he is approaching this interaction. If, for example, Mr. Carvalho elects not to sit on the exam table, this may indicate a certain trepidation with respect to the reason for his visit or for healthcare in general. Perhaps he is uncomfortable being the thing under examination. Making a note of patients' use of the clinical space can therefore offer avenues to further explore when trying to better understand patients' motivations, hesitations, or other concerns.

As the example with Mr. Carvalho demonstrates, even the use of a single chair can communicate a great deal to the patient and the clinician—so too can the overall layout and design of the exam room itself. Below is a visualization of a typical exam room, complete with exam table, companion chairs, clinician workstation, and hanging stethoscope and blood pressure cuff. The ubiquity of this setup has, to some extent, made it the default design for many clinical spaces. But when we interrogate the assumptions guiding this design, and how the nonverbal element of artifactual communication influences both information transmission and the relationship-building components of communication, we learn that a single exam room, indeed, has much to say.

Artifactual communication refers to the phenomenon of how various artifacts—from the clothing or jewelry one wears to the manner of their dress or the style of their hair, to the objects in a room—all convey meaning, whether intentional or unintentional (Burgoon et al., 2021). Looking at the Figure 4.4 depiction

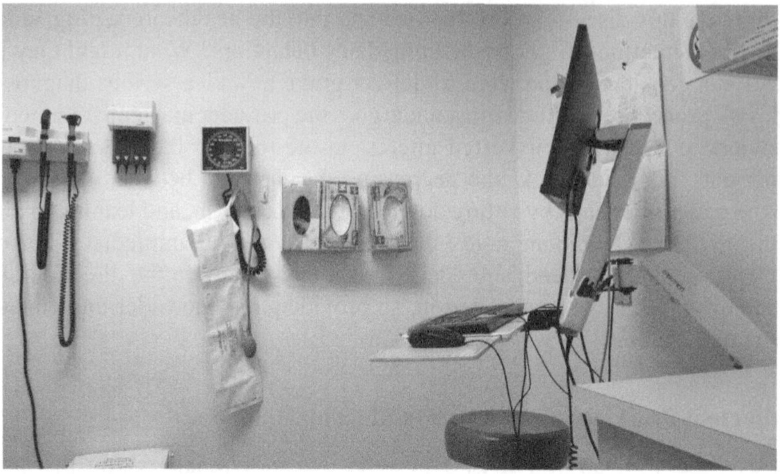

Figure 4.4 A typical exam room. Photo from Shutterstock.

of a typical exam room design, we can reflect on what this layout conveys. In line with a conventional setup, the provider's workstation faces the wall so that as they are interacting with the patient chart, their back would be turned toward the patient. With regard to the report function of communication, this configuration presents obvious barriers to comprehension, as the provider would be projecting their voice away from the patient and any accompanying facial expressions would likewise be obscured from the patient's line of sight. From the perspective of rapport, specifically, having one's back turned to another is symbolically loaded and works to potentially undermine all that is conveyed by the immediacy behaviors described above.

So, this begs the question, "What is a provider to do under such constraints?" One method for engaging with the exam room design is by waiting to chart until after the patient has finished providing their account. It is worth acknowledging, however, that there are merits to charting while the patient is speaking, as the medical literature has documented its added benefit of signaling to the patient that they are actively listening, and, in turn, recording what they are describing (see Duke et al., 2013; Lee et al., 2016). Another way that the provider can engage with the artifacts in the room to facilitate both report and rapport includes performing the exam on the exam table and then inviting them to have a seat in the chair adjacent to the workstation for the consultation part of the visit. This configuration would allow the provider to maintain eye contact and for their facial expressions to be clearly observable throughout the course of the visit. This clearly works in the interest of fostering a productive provider-patient relationship, but also works to draw a symbolic dividing line between the exam portion of the visit and the consultation, thereby signaling a shift from physical assessment to relational meaning making.

So, what else is a simple exam room capable of communicating? Case 2 illustrates how certain design elements embedded within clinical spaces can contribute to, or undermine, cultures of belongingness within medicine. More specifically, Case 2 offers commentary on how artifacts—from a provider's white coat to an elevated, reclined exam table—may signal who such spaces were designed for and who they were not.

Case 2

Scenario: Ms. Landry arrives at a newly renovated outpatient multi-specialty clinic, located just outside of Los Angeles. The clinic has been hailed as a flagship patient center by the local university medical practice that built it. The space is characterized by a minimalist design, complete with standing-height kiosks for self-check-in, smaller exam rooms to maximize the number of patients that can be roomed, and fixed-height exam tables meant to appear as a departure from the look of traditional exam rooms.

Patient: Ms. Landry is a 42-year-old woman with relapsing-remitting multiple sclerosis. Her disease is typically well controlled and she ambulates independently but occasionally uses forearm crutches when her symptoms become less well managed. Her last acute relapse was nine months ago, requiring oral corticosteroid treatment.

Provider: Dr. Williams is a new attending physician, who just graduated from her fellowship program the year prior. Aware of her young age, she is nervous about being seen by patients as a competent physician, and so makes it a point to wear her white coat, with her badge clearly displayed and stethoscope draped around her neck. As a Black woman, she takes pride in wearing her hair naturally, but has fixed it in a tight, low bun.

This is her initial visit with Ms. Landry. While she is running on schedule, she is concerned about efficiently completing the intake documentation efficiently. She walks into the room confidently and cheerfully, and after engaging in routine pleasantries, she asks Ms. Landry to "hop up onto the exam table." Mrs. Landry, looking at the exam table, which is elevated to above hip-level for her, responds, "I'll try my best."

The interaction among Ms. Landry, Dr. Williams, and the clinical space exemplifies how artifactual communication is at work here. Mrs. Landry's hesitance about her ability to "hop up" to an exam table that is at a fixed height underscores the importance of **universal design**. Robert Mace (1998), founder of the Center for Universal Design, defines the concept as "the design of products and environments to be usable by all people, to the greatest extent possible, without the need for adaptation or specialized design" (p. 1). With this definition in mind, one can see how the artifactual communication fostered by the clinic as it is presented above violates the tenets of universal design. The self-guided check-in kiosks, for example, assumes not only that the patient possesses the digital literacy needed to navigate these systems, but that they have the mobility and visual abilities to interact with the touchscreen interface. Furthermore, the smaller exam rooms, while meant to maximize efficiency, may prevent wheelchair users from adequately accessing and navigating this space. Finally, as the above interaction with Mrs. Landry shows, fixed-height exam tables, though perhaps more aesthetically pleasing, are functionally problematic for patients with mobility issues. Universal design would, however, address many of these concerns in that rather than design spaces for use by the majority of users (i.e., able-bodied patients), it generates spaces that may be used *universally*—that is, by all.

In terms of how the artifacts in a particular space impact the patient-provider relationships, one only has to look as far as Ms. Landry's response to Dr. Williams. While it is unlikely that she would have interpreted Dr. Williams' invitation to "hop onto" the exam table as insensitive or indifferent to her limited mobility, such a statement, when taken in conjunction with room layout itself, may inadvertently signal that this space was not made with people like her in mind. Such a feeling of exclusion or isolation is, in turn, bound to negatively impact the provider-patient as a whole (i.e., the rapport shared between them) and consequently influence the nature and volume of the information the patient feels comfortable disclosing (i.e., what they report).

On the subject of belongingness, however, it is not always the patient who questions if they are represented and considered within certain professional spheres. Dr. Williams' deliberate styling of her self-presentation indicates this much. Dr. Williams' decision to wear her white coat, stethoscope, and badge clearly visible may be regarded as her attempt to not be mistaken as something other than a physician. This may stem from a combination of her new status as an attending and as someone who is no longer in training, but it may also be derived from her position as a Black woman in medicine—a demographic that has historically been underrepresented within the field (Lett et al., 2018). In fact, the thought she has put into what her hair might communicate presumably reflects a degree of self-awareness in this regard, especially considering that Black women wearing their hair in natural styles—for example, afros, natural curls, or braids—have often been deemed "unprofessional" in a coded discourse of racism and exclusion (see Opie and Phillips, 2015).

But deliberations over how personal presentation and attire convey who we are to others, and who we want to see us as—what Chapter 3 refers to as avowed and ascribed identities, respectively—extend even farther. Surgeons, for example, often don scrubs, not just for utility, but to symbolically insert themselves in a class of providers. Outpatient sports medicine and orthopedic providers, however, may alternatively opt for a more athletically coded look, wearing elevated "athleisure" attire. Even pediatric ICU nurses, who select "Snoopy" or "Mickey" scrubs, are attempting to fashion a professional identity for themselves, whether that be a "kid-friendly practitioner," "a child at heart," or what have you. Regardless of the specific example under consideration, though, what remains consistent across settings or specialties is that providers of all kinds are constantly engaged in this type of communication, whether they realize it or not.

When considered in its entirety, Case 2 highlights the fact that communication is never neutral, and that it is highly consequential. The environment as it has been manufactured, the technological interfaces embedded within it, and the presentation of the professionals working within the clinic all actively shape how care is relationally maintained and informationally exchanged. When clinical spaces, and the artifacts featured within them are implemented without accounting for the principles of universal design, the patient-provider rapport is placed at risk, as such may subtly communicate exclusion, misrepresentation, or a general lack of belonging. At the same time, these artifacts impact the report function of communication, as patients' willingness to divulge personal information, ask questions, or express concerns depends upon feeling both physically accommodated and socially acknowledged.

Given the importance of the report and rapport as they have thus been outlined in the context of nonverbal communication as a whole, a natural next question asks how one goes about facilitating both functions in concrete clinical contexts. We treat this question as a guiding one in the next section and the specific case presented therein.

Methods for Facilitating Report and Building Rapport

Case 3

Scenario: Ms. Alvarez arrives at a busy primary care clinic for her 3:00 pm appointment. In order to help keep providers on schedule and streamline the intake process, the clinic has kiosks set up in the lobby (such as that featured in Figure 4.5). Ms. Alvarez, frustrated with inputting her data over and over again, offers brief responses only.

Patient: Ms. Alvarez is a 46-year-old woman presenting with chronic fatigue and episodic tightness in her chest. She has been seen by multiple providers for these issues. Despite an extensive work up, no cause has been found for her symptoms. Today, she is also concerned about difficulty sleeping over the past several months.

Provider: Dr. Nguyen is a family medicine physician with 25+ years of experience practicing. She begins the consultation with Ms. Alvarez by pulling up a stool, so that she faces directly in front of Ms. Alvarez. Before reviewing her history, Dr. Nguyen simply asks Ms. Alvarez what has brought her in today. While Ms. Alvarez is speaking, she says little, only nodding her head

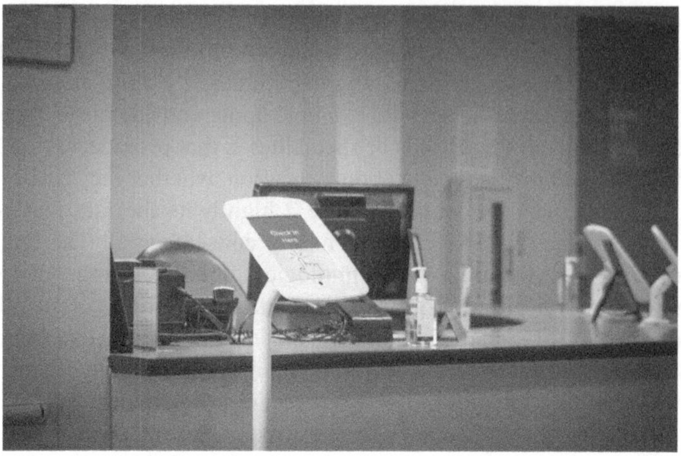

Figure 4.5 A check-in kiosk in a clinic waiting room. Photo from Shutterstock.

> or remarking with the occasional "uh huh" or "mm." Ms. Alvarez eventually goes on to disclose that she is under incredible stress at work and is feeling the weight of caring for both her adolescent children and her aging parents.

Dr. Nguyen discloses that she was in a similar "sandwich" caregiving role—providing care for both her children and parents—and could relate to the stress it causes. She has further history questions and performs an appropriate physical exam. With no concerning findings in the history or in the exam, Dr. Nguyen suspects the symptoms might be psychologic. She then proposes pursuing psychological support in conjunction with a prescription for the short-term hydroxyzine.

Ms. Alvarez expresses concern that she doesn't want to get addicted to "sleeping pills." Dr. Nguyen validates her concern by saying that it is reasonable to be cautious and that she doesn't want that for her either. She explains that hydroxyzine is a non-addictive sleep aid, which, originally prescribed as an anti-itch medication designed to treat allergic reactions, its off-label use has come to include as a sleep aid. Dr. Nguyen pauses to explain that "off label" means that while a medication was not necessarily approved to treat a certain condition, clinicians have found it safe and effective to do so.

> Think of it as using a tool already in our toolbox. For instance, a hammer is typically used to drive in nails, but occasionally, we might also use it to help loosen a stuck board. This medication is operating in the same way.

Dr. Nguyen asks Ms. Alvarez outright if this explanation made sense, to which Ms. Alvarez responds, "Yes, thank you." Dr. Nguyen closes by asking,

"What kinds of questions do you have?" Ms. Alvarez appears to think for a while, not saying anything for several seconds. Ms. Alvarez indicates that she doesn't, and then Dr. Nguyen asks Ms. Alvarez to briefly recount the treatment plan as she understands it.

In analyzing this interaction, it is perhaps most helpful to start at the beginning. One of the first things Dr. Nguyen does upon entering the exam room is pull up a chair so as to be eye-level with Ms. Alvarez. Doing so subtly alters the rapport dynamics between the two, as it both figuratively and literally places the patient and provider on equal footing. Consider the message this communicates when compared to interviewing a patient laying on an exam table while standing over them. Aligning one's feet, knees, hips, shoulders, and head in the direction of their object of interest—here, the patient—can further signal that the provider is granting the patient their undivided interest. The same can be said for reserving charting for after or at the close of visit, rather than while the patient is speaking, like Dr. Nguyen presumably does.

Another thing that Dr. Nguyen does to convey attentiveness, and to thereby facilitate both the report and rapport functions of communication, is through the use of **back-channeling** devices. Back-channeling involves the use of minimal responses like "uh huh," "hm," or "yeah" to indicate both that the interlocutor is listening and attentive, and to implicitly instruct the other party to continue. Popular belief often characterizes these sorts of interjections as harmful interruptions that are disrespectful in that they are perceived to redirect the conversational floor to the one offering such responses. Many scholars of communication, however, denounce this antagonistic view of back-channeling in interaction, instead seeing such contributions as fundamentally cooperative (Schegloff, 1982; Tannen, 2005). For them, the use of such devices is akin to saying, "I'm listening. Keep going!"

Another particularly instructive moment in this case comes when Dr. Nguyen shares with Ms. Alvarez that she had personally experienced the burdens of a dual-caregiving role as well. Professional wisdom has it that the divulgence of personal details such as this by a provider is frowned upon, with some even considering it a breach of their role. However, **social penetration theory**—a well-established paradigm of relational communication—contends that it is through mutual disclosure that the distance between two people is shortened (Altman & Taylor, 1973). Within the field of medicine, specifically, researchers like Beach et al. (2004) identified a variety of functions that physician self-disclosure serves, from providing reassurance to helping the patient extend the narrative of their illness, to building rapport, as we've shown here. The authors also noted that their study of more than 1,000 routine office visits indicated that physician self-disclosure was consistently associated with higher patient satisfaction. Given these findings, providers may consider engaging in a form of self-disclosure akin to what Dr. Nguyen has done here for the purposes of relationship-building with patients.

Shifting our attention briefly to the other side of the patient-provider dynamic—the report function of communication—it is worth noting Dr. Nguyen's use of analogies in the interest of patient comprehension. By comparing off-label use to how one may use the same tool to perform different tasks, Dr. Nguyen is fulfilling the goals of plain language initiatives, as she seeks to compare something unknown to the patient (i.e., the term "off-label") to something known to them (i.e., household tools).

The use of analogies in medicine is a common practice for precisely this reason. That said, a word of caution should be introduced here. In *Illness and Its Metaphors*, Susan Sontag (1978) writes, "The most truthful way of regarding illness—and the healthiest way of being ill—is one most purified of, most resistant to, metaphoric thinking" (p. 3). In Sontag's view, what makes metaphor troublesome is its implications or entailments. Take the commonly used militaristic metaphor that portrays cancer, for instance, as a battle to be won or lost. Such a characterization is evident in statements like, "She won the battle against cancer" or "The disease is attacking his immune system." Sontag argues that while these metaphors may seem innocuous, they create clear winners and losers, and those who fail to overcome the disease just did not "fight" hard enough. Therefore, in taking into account Sontag's position, the use of metaphor in medicine should be done carefully. When employing a metaphor or analogy as Dr. Nguyen does, it would be wise to consider the implications of such.

On the topic of using plain language in clinical encounters, a counterargument must also be considered for completely eschewing jargon. While there may be merit in avoiding jargon or the excessive use of medical terminology when interfacing with patients, some have asserted the utility of "medicalese" in standardizing communication across specialties. According to this view, such standardization facilitates coordinated care because of the precision afforded when everyone "speaks the same language." In their 2021 study of standardized terminologies within nursing and midwifery, for instance, Fennelly et al. found that the use of such language (which may otherwise be dubbed "jargon") exerted a positive impact on communication, quality of care, and interoperability. So, rather than eliminating jargon altogether, a provider may consider "**code-switching**," a process by which they intentionally shift from one manner of speaking, such as in highly specialized terms, to another, such as plain language. This is what Hadden et al. (2018) advocate in their article, "The Bilingual Physician: Seamless Switching from Medicalese to Plain Language." Recognizing the aforementioned value of jargon for certain purposes, the authors encourage providers to "code-switch" from medicalese to plain language when interacting with patients in order to account for varying levels of health literacy.

From Case 3, we can also glean instructive insights regarding question-and-answer sequences. It is noteworthy that Dr. Nguyen asks, "What kinds of questions do you have?" instead of "Do you have questions?" The former of these questions is open-ended, meaning that they prompt the patient to respond in a more detailed manner, beyond a one-word yes/no reply. The latter of these phrasings, however, is structured so as to be answered with a single-word response, and therefore, is comparatively less adept at encouraging the patient to elaborate upon any areas where they may be confused, aspects of their care where they lack comprehension, or areas where they still harbor reservations. Therefore, in this regard, a thoughtful phrasing of such questions may work in the interest of the report function of communication in that it carves out a deliberate space within the interaction for the patient to detail their concerns in more than just a word or two.

Acknowledging and allowing for extended periods of silence work in much the same way. Referring to the details of Case 3 as they are presented above, the patient, Ms. Alvarez, remains silent for several seconds after Dr. Nguyen has explained the safety of the medication she is prescribing. When viewing the interaction from the outside, this may appear unremarkable. However, in practice, it is very difficult to permit prolonged, uninterrupted silence. In fact, *Time Magazine* (2010) noted this in their story headlined, "Awkward Silence: 4 Seconds Is All It Takes to Feel Rejected." The authors ground this claim in a study by Koudenburg et al. (2011), who argue that even brief periods of silence disrupt the conversational flow, and such flow is "associated with positive emotions, and a heightened sense of belonging, self-esteem, social validation and consensus" (p. 512). The researchers continue that if "a brief silence disrupts this fluency, negative emotions and feelings of rejection arise" (p. 512).

So, what does this mean in the context of the above case and medicine in general? It may mean that silence in conversation must be navigated carefully. Providers should grant patients sufficient interactional space to reflect on the details of their care. However, extended silences may likewise be worth gently pursuing. Does the patient's extended silence communicate confusion or disappointment? Does it signal uncertainty about the proposed plan of care or hesitancy to voice their concerns? Furthermore, how much silence is too much? While it would be ill-advised to universally apply a time limit to any single episode of silence, the findings referenced in the above study may be a helpful starting point. That said, the provider's intuition will likely be their best guide; if the interaction feels stunted, awkward, or otherwise derailed, these momentary pauses can be informative and junctures that serve as opportunities for aligning patient and provider perspectives

A Guide, Not a Prescription, for Communication

While the previous section outlined different aspects of the clinical encounter that may contribute to improved understanding and even a higher quality of care, it stops short of prescribing certain actions to be taken for use in all healthcare scenarios. To do so would be more in line with the transmission view of communication that has thus been problematized both in the academic literature and within this chapter alone. Ultimately, a provider skilled in communication principles and practices would recognize that while certain elements of the interaction may impact the report and rapport functions of communication, they do not determine them. Referring back to the previously discussed aspects of artifactual communication in the clinic, a provider may choose to wear scrubs in an outpatient clinic purely out of comfort and utility, whereas others read this gesture as pompousness—as the provider's attempt to remind other clinic staff that they belong in the surgeon class. As this example shows, even when we have the best intentions, the interaction may not—and often does not—go as planned. However, by accounting for the various elements that impact clinical communication—from the physical layout of the exam room to culturally specific notions of time, to nonverbal gestures—the provider is well-positioned to pivot should the interaction be derailed.

Yet, all of this talk of "the provider" here is somewhat misleading in that it seems to suggest that the burden of effective communication in the clinic falls upon a single individual. The following chapter on organizational communication, however, details how established communication pathways within hospitals, clinics, and so on enable or constrain communication as well. It provides a detailed look into how coordination, and ideally collaboration, among various members of the care team impacts patient care. Thus, the burden of effective communication becomes distributed and the axiom of "One cannot not communicate" may be better thought of as "One cannot not communicate within broader systems of care."

Glossary

- **Rapport**
- **Report**
- **Transmission model of communication**
- **Psychological noise**
- **Physiological noise**
- **Agency**
- **Constitutive model of communication**
- **Chronemics**
- **Monochronic**
- **Polychronic**
- **Proxemics**
- **High-contact cultures**
- **Artifactual communication**
- **Universal design**
- **Back-channeling**
- **Social penetration theory**
- **Code-switching**

Exercises

1. For this exercise, you will take an artifactual inventory. What does your presentation of self say about you? What are you trying to convey to others, both intentionally and perhaps unintentionally? How might this influence clinical interactions?
2. Sketch a design for the ideal exam room. What makes it ideal? What do the various elements included in the room communicate to patients and providers?

Further Reading

- To learn more about plain language initiatives in medicine, visit the CDC's relevant page: https://www.cdc.gov/health-literacy/php/develop-materials/plain-language.html
- To learn more about using plain language for patients with low health literacy, visit the NIH's website here: https://www.nih.gov/institutes-nih/nih-office-director/office-communications-public-liaison/clear-communication/clear-simple

References

Adler, R. B., Rodman, G., & du Pré, A. (2020). *Understanding human communication* (14th ed.). Oxford University Press.

Altman, I., & Taylor, D. A. (1973). *Social penetration: The development of interpersonal relationships*. Holt, Rinehart & Winston.

Baile, W. F., Buckman, R., Lenzi, R., Glober, G., Beale, E. A., & Kudelka, A. P. (2000). SPIKES—a six-step protocol for delivering bad news: Application to the patient with cancer. *The Oncologist*, *5*(4), 302–311.

Beach, M. C., Roter, D., Rubin, H., Frankel, R., Levinson, W., & Ford, D. E. (2004). Is physician self-disclosure related to patient evaluation of office visits? *Journal of General Internal Medicine*, *19*(9), 905–910.

Burgoon, J. K., Guerrero, L. K., & Floyd, K. (2021). *Nonverbal communication* (2nd ed.). Routledge.

Craig, R. T. (1999). Communication theory as a field. *Communication Theory*, *9*(2), 119–161.

Duke, P., Frankel, R. M., & Reis, S. (2013). How to integrate the electronic health record and patient-centered communication into the medical visit: A skills-based approach. *Teaching and Learning in Medicine*, *25*(4), 358–365.

Fennelly, O., Grogan, L., Reed, A., & Hardiker, N. R. (2021). Use of standardized terminologies in clinical practice: A scoping review. *International Journal of Medical Informatics*, *149*, 104431.

Hadden, K., Coleman, C., & Scott, A. (2018). The bilingual physician: Seamless switching from Medicalese to plain language. *Journal of Graduate Medical Education*, *10*(2), 130–133.

Hall, E. T. (1959). *The silent language*. Doubleday.

Koudenburg, N., Postmes, T., & Gordijn, E. H. (2011). Disrupting the flow: How brief silences in group conversations affect social needs. *Journal of Experimental Social Psychology*, *47*(2), 512–515.

Lee, W. W., Alkureishi, M. A., Ukabiala, O., Venable, L. R., Ngooi, S. S., Staisiunas, D. D., & Arora, V. M. (2016). Patient perceptions of electronic medical record use by faculty and resident physicians: A mixed methods study. *Journal of General Internal Medicine*, *31*(11), 1315–1322.

Lett, E., Orji, W. U., & Sebro, R. (2018). Declining racial and ethnic representation in clinical academic medicine: A longitudinal study of 16 US medical specialties. *PLoS One*, *13*(11), e0207274.

Littlejohn, S. W & Foss, K. A. (Eds.). (2009). *Encyclopedia of communication theory* (Vols. 1–2). Sage Publications.

Mace, R. L. (1998). Universal design in housing. *Assistive Technology*, *10*(1), 21–28. https://doi.org/10.1080/10400435.1998.10131957

Mehrabian, A. (1971). *Silent messages*. Wadsworth Publishing.

Opie, T. R., & Phillips, K. W. (2015). Hair penalties: The negative influence of Afrocentric hair on ratings of Black women's dominance and professionalism. *Frontiers in Psychology*, *6*, 311.

Schegloff, E. A. (1982). Discourse as an interactional achievement: Some uses of "uh huh" and other things that come between sentences. In D. Tannen (Ed.), *Analyzing discourse: Text and talk* (pp. 71–93). Georgetown University Press.

Shannon, C. E., & Weaver, W. (1949). *The mathematical theory of communication*. University of Illinois Press.

Sontag, S. (1978). *Illness as metaphor*. Farrar, Strauss & Giroux.

Tannen, D. (2005). *Conversational style: Analyzing talk among friends*. Oxford University Press.

Watzlawick, P., Beavin, J. B., & Jackson, D. D. (1967). *Pragmatics of human communication: A study of interactional patterns, pathologies, and paradoxes*. W. W. Norton & Company.

Wittenberg, E., Ferrell, B., Goldsmith, J., Ragan, S. L., & Paice, J. (2016). Assessment of a statewide palliative care team training course: COMFORT communication for palliative care teams. *Journal of Palliative Medicine*, *19*(7), 746–752.

5 Communicating within Organizations

Hierarchies, Handoffs, and the Hidden Curriculum

The White Coat as a Symbol of Medical Hierarchy

The elusive white coat is one of the most salient symbols of the medical training journey (see Figure 5.1). Once only extended to medical students who graduated from medical school, this symbol of the beginning of a successful medical education has since been adopted by a variety of other health professions, including nurse practitioners, physician assistants, and pharmacists. Students in training for each of these health professions are often conveyed the white coat via the longstanding organizational ritual of the white coat ceremony. Yet, at the ceremony, which usually takes place during their first year of training, new matriculants are issued a white coat several inches shorter than what might be considered standard. At least in the case of medical doctor (MD) and doctor of osteopathic medicine (DO) programs, the full-length white coat—the white coat so many associate with doctors—is not granted to students until after graduation, around the time that they enter residency.

Why do this? Why create a "trainee" version of the white coat and reserve the full-length artifact for those who have completed their training? The short answer is to distinguish students from those with greater knowledge and/or experience. The white coat serves as a symbolic distinction to others (patients, fellow providers, and other members of the care team) denoting their trainee status, but perhaps more importantly, it offers a similar reminder to the student themselves. It reminds them of the activities, interactions, and modes of communication available to them as students, and those that are not. In short, it signals their place within the well-established medical hierarchy.

The hierarchical structure of medicine is a defining feature of medical education. It defines who reports to whom, and in doing so, prescribes communication pathways. The well-entrenched nature of these organizational hierarchies and the effects they have on healthcare communication are precisely why medical hierarchies represent the first part of this three-part chapter. Case 1 examines how superiority and subordination impact the reporting of uncertainties and impede the free flow of information so as to ultimately affect patient health.

DOI: 10.4324/9781003654308-5

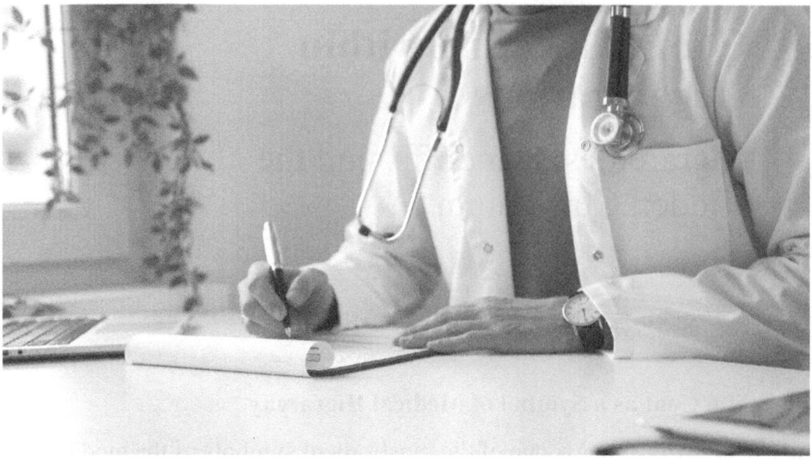

Figure 5.1 A physician wearing a white coat and stethoscope. Photo from Shutterstock.

It considers the possibility of lateral communication, and in step with contemporary theories of communication (i.e., the Communicative Constitution of Organization (CCO) perspective) how restructuring the pathways of communication may ultimately reconstitute the hierarchies themselves.

The second part of this three-part chapter considers how these hierarchies, as well as time constraints and institutional routines, impact a key juncture of healthcare communication: patient handoffs. Referring to the transfer of a patient's care from one provider to another, **handoffs** are a site of frequent communication breakdown. In transitioning care from one provider to another, questions arise as to what information is being included, what is being left out, and whose voice is treated as authoritative.

Finally, the third part of this chapter, as represented by Case 3, examines the hidden curriculum of medical education. While the "hidden" in "hidden curriculum" may suggest, for some, intentional duplicitous or other ulterior motives, what it actually signifies is all that providers-in-training are taught through less formal means. Rather than be delivered in classrooms, lecture halls, and labs, this curriculum is imparted in hallways, breakrooms, and even, as the following chapter will show, through coded language in the patient's chart. And instead of this curriculum being conveyed through overt means and formal teachings, it is communicated in the most unsuspecting of ways—in jokes, in offhand comments, and in subtle corrections to a perceived transgression.

Case 1 begins by examining how organizational hierarchies within medicine impact the quality of the care being provided. It explores these hierarchies both among physicians and medical students, as well as across interprofessional contexts (with nurses, technicians, and other members of the care team). It is worth mentioning, however, that while Case 1 engages with the concept of organizational hierarchies in a more explicit manner, such hierarchies provide the backdrop for each of the cases presented in this chapter. These discrete yet integrated cases therefore serve as steppingstones to the chapter's conclusion, which argues that the organizational culture in which communication occurs matters just as much as the content of that communication.

Case 1

Patient: Mr. Samuel Carter is a 70-year-old African American man admitted to the hospital of a large academic medical center in Baltimore, Maryland (U.S.) with shortness of breath (Figure 5.2). He has a history of chronic obstructive pulmonary disease (COPD) and heart failure. In the past year, he has been hospitalized twice, once for pneumonia and once for hypervolemia. In just the past few hours, he has increasingly required more oxygen, going from two to four liters.

Providers: Mr. Carter's care team consists of Dr. Priyanka Patel, an intern in her first year of residency; Dr. Michael Porter, a senior resident in the third year of residency; Dr. Melissa Timmerman, the attending physician on service; and Maria Dela Cruz, the nurse caring for Mr. Carter for the past three shifts as well as his two prior admissions.

Scenario: During morning rounds, Dr. Patel presents the patient, saying, "Mr. Carter is a 70-year-old male with COPD and CHF admitted for suspected pneumonia. His oxygen requirements have doubled over night. I'm concerned that fluid overload may be a contributing factor, though worsening infection is also a–"

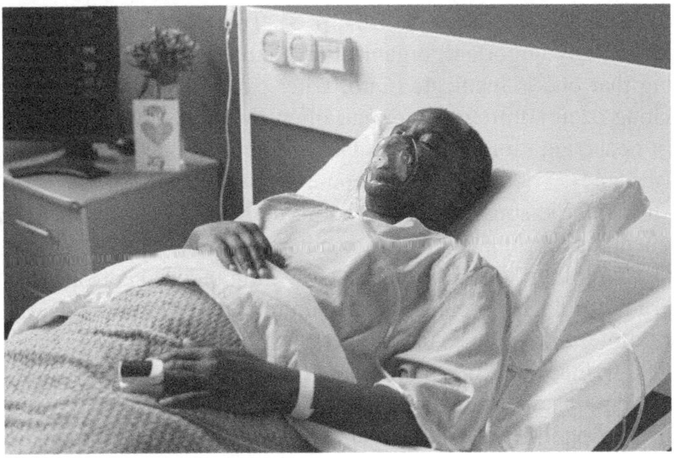

Figure 5.2 A patient receiving oxygen support. Photo from iStock.

> Before Dr. Patel can finish her assessment, Dr. Timmerman interjects, "You need to speak like someone who has had eight years of education. If you think it's fluid overload, then just say that."
>
> Dr. Patel begins again: "Mr. Carter's symptoms are most consistent with heart failure exacerbation."
>
> Dr. Timmerman nods in seeming approval and recommends upping the dosage of diuretics.
>
> A few hours later, Maria approaches the team, saying, "I'm not sure it's due to fluid overload. In the past, when he's experiencing fluid overload, we see pronounced swelling and rapid weight gain. We're just not seeing that here. And when his infection has worsened, we tend to see his breathing deteriorate like this."
>
> Dr. Porter responds, "We've already put in the order for the diuretics. Let's just keep an eye on it."
>
> By 7:00 pm, Mr. Carter becomes hypotensive and his lab results return, indicating sepsis. The team decides to discontinue the diuretics and start antibiotics.

While this episode may appear extreme in its treatment of Dr. Patel and Nurse Dela Cruz, as well as its portrayal of Drs. Porter and Timmerman as anything from dismissive to downright condescending, it is not atypical in the broader history of organizational culture within medicine. Just as a society can be said to have a culture typified by its own set of beliefs, values, shared languages, rituals, symbols, and daily practices, the same can be said for medicine. **Organizational culture** may be defined as "a pattern of shared basic assumptions learned by a group as it solved its problems of external adaptation and internal integration, that has worked well enough to be considered valid and, therefore, to be taught" (Schein, 1984, p. 3). The latter part of Schein's definition is particularly important: organizational culture is something that is taught, something that one is inculcated into. Later parts of this chapter address how this teaching occurs through informal, often overlooked, means, but here, one can see it occurring more overtly as Dr. Timmerman openly chastises Dr. Patel for her hesitancy. Therefore, in the context of this definition of organizational culture, this interpersonal exchange is not necessarily the result of individual temperament or workplace relations, but rather reflective of a longstanding "way of doing things" (teaching included) within medical education.

And truth be told, the organizational culture of many medical institutions was, for a long time, a toxic one. In fact, up until the 1980s, it was not uncommon for medical trainees to work more than 100 hours per week. This is where the term "resident" came from; doctors completing their residency quite literally lived at the hospital. Early adopters of this arrangement, like the medical education program at Johns Hopkins University in Baltimore, MD (where this case is set), found that housing residents on site offered many advantages, most notable among which is that they could be perpetually on call. For the residents, though, this meant giving up a life that existed outside of the hospital. This all changed, however, in 1984 with the death of Libby Zion at a New York teaching hospital. An 18-year-old college student, Zion, was admitted for fever and agitation. She was administered meperidine but was already taking a monoamine oxidase inhibitor, a combination later believed to have contributed to serotonin syndrome and later, cardiac arrest. Zion's father argued that her death was the result of medical error stemming from overworked residents. His advocacy eventually led to legislation in the form of the 1989 Libby Zion law, which capped resident working hours at 80 hours per week (Poulose et al., 2005). The Accreditation Council for Graduate Medical Education (ACGME) followed suit shortly thereafter in 2003 by applying similar standards across the nation (Nasca et al., 2010).

The Zion case demonstrates the tangible dangers brought to patient health as a result of negative organizational culture, but it is worth pointing out that organizational cultures do not exist in a vacuum. Organizational cultures exist within larger cultures and the boundaries separating the organization from the broader culture in which it is situated are fundamentally permeable. Within the context of the New York teaching hospital referenced above, this means that the hospital itself was influenced by both the working norms of medicine and the U.S. as a whole. In the U.S., long working hours and measurable self-sacrifice have been equated with dedication to one's professional role and moral stamina. Sociologists refer to this phenomenon as the "work devotion schema," wherein those remaining constantly available to employers and persisting amidst grueling working conditions are imbued with greater societal value (Williams, 2001). Against this broader cultural backdrop, then, grueling residencies, toxic organizational cultures, and "tough love" approaches to medical education were considered a sign of both professional strength and seriousness. And while the work devotion schema may be especially prevalent in the U.S., it is not unique to American culture. This is why oversight bodies in the European Union have passed similar initiatives in the form of the Working Time Directive, which specified a 48-hour maximum work week for physicians across 48 member states (European Parliament & Council of the European Union, 2003).

While these formal mechanisms put into place to combat the effects of an organizational culture predicated on overworking healthcare personnel represent a step in the right direction, they alone do not entirely address the problem at hand. In both the U.S. and the E.U., the primary method for tracking medical trainee working hours is through self-report. These reported logs are then submitted for review to program directors, but ample research has shown that residents consistently underreport the number of hours worked. For example, in their survey of 26,581 residents, Drolet et al. (2013) found that nearly half of these individuals (42.9%) reported falsely documenting their duty hours at some time. This invites the question of why so many medical trainees feel the need to underreport their working hours. One possible explanation lies in how perceptions of self-worth are tied to excessive work, as described above. Another explanation, however, lies in an organizational culture that conveys, albeit implicitly (through a hidden curriculum), that this is both a norm and an expectation of graduate medical education. Accurately reporting duty hours may therefore feel like a violation of such cultural norms, as would Dr. Patel's speaking up, given the well-established medical education hierarchy that follows an intern → resident → senior or chief resident → attending format (see Figure 5.3).

It should be noted that there are ways that medical hierarchy can be helpful. A less experienced student can learn from an intern who is just a year or two more experienced. For similar reasons, an intern can learn from a more advanced resident, a resident from a fellow, a fellow from an attending, and a new attending from a more experienced colleague. Medical care is complex, and in the best case scenario, the medical hierarchy can gradually introduce appropriate tasks and knowledge in a staggered fashion. This can allow a trainee to become gradually more independent, in the confines of a safe, collaborative team environment. The benefits of hierarchy can also play out in medical care between professions in medicine.

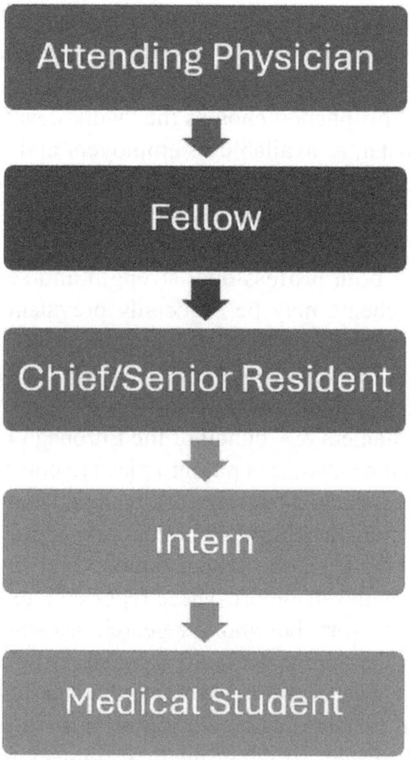

Figure 5.3 An organizational hierarchy of medical staff. Image is author-generated

The skills and work of a medical assistant can offload the work of a nurse. The nurse of a patient can filter the important questions and data to the physician. This is why in contemporary medical organizations, a primary goal of the organization is to allow the benefits of the medical hierarchy to persist while mitigating its risks.

Groupthink, Spirals of Silence, and Cost of Consensus

Indeed, it is the organizational culture of a particular institution and medicine in general that makes some members of the care team feel safe to voice their concerns even—and especially—when they go against general consensus. An organizational culture that penalizes speaking up and speaking "out of turn" (i.e., in a manner that does not adhere to prescribed organizational hierarchies) is unlikely to see practitioners like Dr. Patel and Nurse Dela Cruz persist in proposing alternative diagnoses. This presents especially detrimental impacts for diagnostic accuracy, especially when one considers that speaking out against the majority view is a protective measure against **groupthink.**

A term coined by the American psychologist Irving Janis (1972), "groupthink" refers to a process in which members of a team or organization prioritize unanimity over the "realistic appraisal of alternatives" (Kretchmar, 2021). In his research, Janis identified groupthink as a primary reason behind poor decision-making, citing high-profile cases of this psychological phenomenon like the Bay of Pigs debacle, the *Challenger* explosion, and the escalation of the Vietnam War. And while Janis offered several plausible explanations as to why groupthink occurs, a select few are particularly relevant to the analysis of Case 1.

One of the primary reasons groupthink occurs is due to concerns for maintaining group harmony. So, while both Dr. Patel and Nurse Dela Cruz have reservations about the rest of the care team's assessment, they may resist escalating these concerns out of fear of undermining the cohesion of the team. This may be even more of a concern for Dr. Patel as challenging leadership (here, Drs. Porter and Timmerman) could be perceived as a direct threat to group dynamics. The fact that both Dr. Patel and Nurse Dela Cruz only voice their dissenting opinion once suggests that self-censorship may also be at play here. Self-censorship occurs when members of a group or team refrain from expressing dissenting opinions—or continuing to express them as in Case 1—for fear of judgment or reprisal. They may self-censor due to what Janis refers to as the "illusion of unanimity." Dr. Patel and Nurse Dela Cruz may believe that all other members of the care team (particularly Drs. Porter and Timmerman) are in agreement and therefore do not want to be the "odd one out," so to speak.

This fear of voicing concerns can, in turn, create what Noelle-Neumann (1974) terms a "spiral of silence." While Noelle-Neumann initially applied this phrase to describe public opinion in mass media settings, its fundamental premise that people suppress opinions that they believe do not reflect the majority view is nonetheless applicable here. This silence then "spirals," compounding and reinforcing the dominant view through the lack of introduction of alternative views challenging it. Noelle-Neumann identifies a fear of social isolation as a primary motivation for remaining silent. When applied to an organizational context—specifically, healthcare—one can see how a fear of social isolation translates to a fear of negative impacts to one's professional advancement. Dr. Patel may not persist with her alternative diagnosis for fear of reprisal; after all, Dr. Timmerman will be evaluating her. Others on the care team, too, implicitly learn what happens when one indicates uncertainty as Dr. Patel did. They witness Dr. Timmerman correct and chastise her, and may therefore internalize that they too should offer a singular diagnosis and resist expressing uncertainty. With this, the silence spirals and as it does, the patient's well-being hangs in the balance.

In this way, both groupthink and the spiral of silence it produces may be seen as working against differential diagnosis. At its core, differential diagnosis operates by considering multiple divergent alternative explanations for a patient's symptoms. It entails producing several plausible explanations and voicing uncertainty as it arises. In the context of Case 1, however, no alternative explanations are entertained, and when they are proffered, they are quickly dismissed in favor of the prevailing hypothesis. Groupthink may therefore be seen as the enemy of diagnostic accuracy, and by extension, patient safety.

When consensus feels inevitable and thus difficult to challenge in team-based settings, and addressing the possibility of error through more informal, conversational means proves insufficient, one may need to turn to more formal reporting mechanisms. Whistleblowing is one such mechanism; it represents one of the last safeguards available for protecting patient safety. Within organizational settings, **whistleblowers** are those individuals who report or otherwise call attention to wrongdoing or neglect. Whistleblowers in healthcare are especially important, given the high-stakes nature of organizational activities, which may quite literally be framed in terms of life and death.

With respect to Case 1, whistleblowing should not be Dr. Patel's and Nurse Dela Cruz's first course of action. This sort of formal reporting is typically reserved for medical negligence or gross misconduct, not diagnostic error. What they can do is first, voice their dissent again. If their dissent is once more dismissed, then they can move up the "chain of command." Nurse Dela Cruz can express her reservations to her charge nurse and Dr. Patel can express them to Dr. Porter.

It is important to acknowledge that the organizational hierarchies typifying medicine did not emerge from nowhere, nor have they endured without some utility. The benefits of a clearly established hierarchical structure is that the communication pathways are unambiguous; every member of the care team knows who they report to. In theory, this means that less important information could be lost as each healthcare professional knows the endpoint of such information (though Case 2 will illustrate the problems that often accompany this transfer of patient information). These hierarchies are also redundant in nature, meaning that the same information gets reviewed by multiple parties—the intern, the resident, the attending, and so on. What this means for the patients is more checkpoints where their diagnoses and treatment plans are being reviewed. In fact, this is one reason why academic medical centers, which feature multi-tiered care teams, have been shown to have reduced patient morbidity and mortality rates, and better health outcomes overall (Burke et al., 2017). All of this is to say that hierarchies are not exclusively bad, but their communicative pitfalls should nonetheless not be ignored.

The question then becomes one of how best to overcome these pitfalls, as they are presented in Case 1. The first course of action is not prescribed for Dr. Patel and Nurse Dela Cruz; it's geared toward Drs. Porter and Timmerman. To counteract the effects of groupthink and preempt a spiral of silence, they can and should actively invite dissent. What might this look like in practice? It may be as simple as asking, "What else could it [the diagnosis] be?" It would entail fully exploring all differential diagnoses, even unlikely ones. And finally, it would reward uncertainty in clinical teaching practices. Perhaps this might be through so simple a comment as, "I appreciate that you are expressing your reservations here. Let's explore this further."

Case 2

Patient: Mrs. Margaret Barnes is a 72-year-old woman recently admitted to a National Health Service (NHS) teaching hospital in Brighton, U.K. She presented with fever (39.1C/102.4F), diffuse abdominal pain, and vomiting. She has a history of Type 2 diabetes, chronic kidney disease, and atrial fibrillation.

Upon being assessed in the Accident & Emergency (A&E) department, imaging from ultrasound and CT suggest acute cholecystitis. She has been admitted for overnight observation, so she can receive intravenous antibiotics while awaiting a surgical consult in the morning.

Overnight, however, Mrs. Barnes' status worsens, as she becomes hypotensive and displays confusion. Her night nurse, Nurse McLean, has also noted decreased urine output. Her fluctuating vital signs thus set an escalation protocol into motion.

Providers: Mrs. Barnes' care is being overseen by multiple clinicians across several shifts. Dr. Fatima Rahman is a Foundation Year 1 physician (i.e., a first-year intern) on the overnight admissions team; Dr. Michael Watson serves as the medical registrar (i.e., a senior resident) overseeing the night team; Dr. Amelia Clarke works the day shift and serves as a consulting physician; Nurse Sean McLean is Mrs. Barnes's night-shift nurse and Nurse Rebecca Greene is her day-time nurse. The general surgery team is scheduled to round on Mrs. Barnes in the morning.

Scenario: At 7:15, the night-shift is preparing for sign-out, during which time Dr. Rahman will hand off care of her patients to the day-time team. She has received multiple complex admissions overnight, meaning that she has a significant amount of information to report in little time.

When it comes time to summarize Mrs. Barnes's condition, she does so in the following manner: "Mrs. Barnes is a 72-year-old woman admitted due to suspected cholecystitis. On antibiotic drip since 13:00. Appeared stable overnight."

Fatigued after multiple admissions overnight, in order to quickly get through her remaining list of patients, Dr. Rahman does not go into detail about other observations she witnessed overnight, including Mrs. Barnes's increased confusion, transient hypotension, and Nurse McLean's report of reduced urine output.

During the separate nurse sign-out and handoff procedure, Nurse McLean informs Nurse Greene of this observation, as well as his interpretations of Mrs. Barnes's condition, saying, "She seems more muddled than when she first arrived. I'm not comfortable calling her 'stable' (Figure 5.4)." Although Nurse McLean shared these concerns with Dr. Rahman, they were interpreted as not warranting escalation at the time and were thus not incorporated into the sign-out report for the incoming care team.

A few hours later, during the ward rounds, Dr. Clarke describes Mrs. Barnes to the rest of the team as "awaiting surgical consult, no urgent concerns at present."

By 12:00, Mrs. Barnes's condition has rapidly deteriorated: she is now hypotensive and unresponsive. Lab results reveal elevated lactate levels, elevated creatinine, and an increasing white blood cell count. Taken together, Ms. Barnes is now in sepsis. She is then immediately transferred to the intensive care unit (ICU) for initiation of IV pressors to reduce end organ damage.

What we see in Case 2 is a communication failure at a critical juncture: the handoff, also referred to as a "handover" in the U.K., where this case is set. It is important to recognize that handoffs are not sites of information transmission (to call back to Chapter 4's discussion of the transmission model of communication); instead, it involves active interpretation and extensive translation work. The reporting clinician must select, interpret, and distill complex information

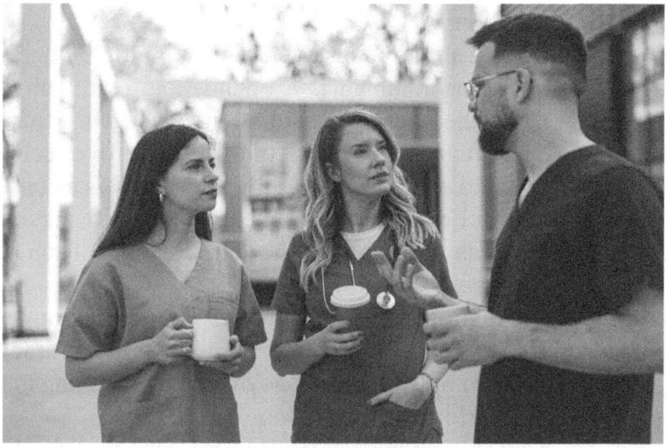

Figure 5.4 Nurses discussing their patient. Image from Shutterstock.

into actionable data. As Eisenberg et al. (2005) point out in their study of communication within the emergency department (ED), these processes of translation necessitate crafting coherent narratives from both fragmented and diverse sources of information. Once this narrative is established, it must once again undergo transformation as it is converted into what the authors term a "technical rationality"—that is, task-oriented information conducive to initiating various actions. Technical rationalities are favored within healthcare organizations because they are often perceived as less ambiguous and messy and more straightforward and decisive than narrative knowledge—knowledge produced and conveyed through patient and provider stories.

The problem, however, as Case 2 illustrates, is that these stories are often important yet full of nuanced health information, and it moreover demonstrates how these nuances can be lost or discarded when they do not easily fit with a technical rationality. For example, when Nurse McLean discloses to Nurse Greene his concerns that he is uncomfortable designating Mrs. Barnes as stable, given what he saw, these observations are largely excluded from the subsequent handoff, not because they are deemed unimportant, but because they do not represent definitive medical realities and are therefore difficult to translate into a technical rationality. In acknowledging organizational preferences for certain kinds of discourses (i.e., specific ways of speaking and describing patients' conditions), we can come to interpret the failure to properly convey this information not as an individual oversight, but as part of broader organizational tendencies to prioritize information characterized by both certainty and actionability.

So, it was not that changes in Mrs. Barnes's condition went unnoticed; it was that they could not be easily framed in clinically actionable terms. Another contributing factor is that this information was confined to two parallel communication systems. It was conveyed within the nursing channel of communication between Nurse McLean and Nurse Greene, and it was separately discussed among Dr. Rahman's team of doctors, though input was derived from Nurse McLean's observations. Medicine has historically kept these two communication channels separate because the workflows, mechanisms of accountability, and various responsibilities of nurses and physicians are inherently different. Nursing emphasizes continuous care and bedside monitoring, whereas physicians focus on formulating their diagnostic reasoning and planning a course of action for medical intervention.

As Case 1 has shown, insights garnered from nursing observations may offer invaluable contextual information that is inherently actionable as physicians attempt to plan their medical interventions. That is why one change organizations like the hospital featured in Case 2 may wish to implement includes working toward making communication among different members of Mrs. Barnes's care team more integrated. Admittedly, conducting joint handoffs where both nursing staff and supervising physicians are present for each and every patient would be logistically difficult. Differing shift start and end times and the fact that physicians cover multiple units makes this unfeasible. What is feasible, however, is more targeted joint discussion. Many hospitals already implement these "safety huddles" for at-risk individuals, such as unstable patients, patients being actively watched/observed, or those who are pending discharge but with concerns (Ghoul et al., 2025). So, one of the members of Mrs. Barnes's care team (e.g., Nurse McLean) could flag her as a patient who might warrant a safety huddle.

Additionally, if differing patient commitments and workloads prohibit in-person safety huddles, different members of the care team can, and should, express concerns in the patient chart. Many existing EMR systems already include fields where these concerns can be documented—by both physicians and nurses. Therefore, implementing changes toward more integrated communication among members of the care team would not necessarily entail large-scale overhauls, but simply leveraging tools already available to them. These tools also allow for healthcare professionals to use language consistent with early warning systems. By using language like "clinician concern" or "staff worried" in the patient EMR, this alone can be sufficient to trigger escalation of rapid response systems, even when the patient's physiological signs appear normal (Sandroni et al., 2007; Williams, 2022).

When these interventions are outlined, what happened to Mrs. Barnes appears more and more preventable. But it also becomes less defined as the negligence of a single individual and rather the result of systemic communication failures. Such failures are pervasive, with data published by the Joint Commission estimating that nearly 70% of **sentinel events**—that is, "a patient safety event that results in death, permanent harm, or severe temporary harm" (Joint Commission, n.d.)—were attributable to communication errors (Dingley et al., 2008). Furthermore, of these medical errors, 80% lied in issues with handoffs (Riesenberg, 2012). Given the scope of the problem, a singular intervention is unlikely to engender significant change. So, what other communication-based tools can one apply under such circumstances? One well-established practice has been used in the airline industry for years: **closed-loop acknowledgment**. Closed-loop acknowledgment occurs when one party restates, paraphrases, or otherwise confirms the information they have received. Commercial airlines have been using this communication system as far back as the 1970s with the initiation of the Crew Resource Management (CRM) system, a training protocol for reducing communication-based errors in aviation (Salas et al., 2006). In practice, closed-loop acknowledgment might look like this:

Pilot: Set flaps to 15.
First Officer: Flaps set to 15.
Pilot: Confirmed.

Here, not only does the first-officer repeat back the information they have received, thus offering the opportunity for correcting any misunderstandings, in the last turn, the pilot confirms that this reporting back of information has been received, effectively "closing the loop" of communication.

Aviation and healthcare share a great deal in common. They are both high-stakes settings, where the lives of multiple individuals are on the line. In both settings, decisions must be made from input from several different personnel, whether that be pilots, flight attendants, and air traffic control in the context of aviation, or physicians, nurses, and support staff within healthcare. Furthermore, both settings feature moments of acute crises, meaning that decisions must be made quickly, often with incomplete information. That is why the closed-loop communication that has proven so effective within commercial aviation has direct implications for healthcare. That said, what might closed-loop communication look like in Case 2? See below for an example closed-loop exchange between Dr. Rahman and Nurse McLean.

Nurse McLean:	Mrs. Barnes looked a little out of it last night. There's also the matter of her urine output dropping. I don't think we can label her stable.
Dr. Rahman:	So I'm hearing that you're worried that she may be deteriorating even though her vitals are stable. Is that right?
Nurse McLean:	Yes, that's right.
Dr. Rahman:	Okay, let's flag her for a safety huddle in the morning.

Within this brief exchange, we see the closed-loop protocol be implemented to effectively translate Nurse McLean's narrative rationality (i.e., his observations) into a technical one (i.e., an actionable next step in the form of the safety huddle). We see Dr. Rahman report back the information she has received, wait for Nurse McLean to confirm its accuracy, and then close the communication loop.

Another final intervention point that this exchange demonstrates is a future orientation. Typically, handoffs involve a reporting of *what is* rather than what *might become*. There is acknowledgment that Mrs. Barnes's present condition is technically stable but also a looking to the future as to how this might change and need to be reassessed: "let's flag her for a safety huddle in the morning."

While these interventions for addressing communication breakdowns in handoffs can be taught outright, there is a great deal in medicine that is learned more informally. Yet, just because this knowledge is implicitly acquired, this does not mean that it is any less salient or that it has any less bearing on one's practice. Case 3 dives into some of these more informal learnings, exploring their various sources and how they ultimately impact patient health.

Case 3

Patient: Mr. Daniel Morales is a 46-year-old man presenting to the ED of a large urban academic medical center located in the Northeastern U.S. (Figure 5.5). He complains of severe back pain, describing it as "excruciating" and rating his pain level a 10 out of 10. He reports that the pain began earlier that same

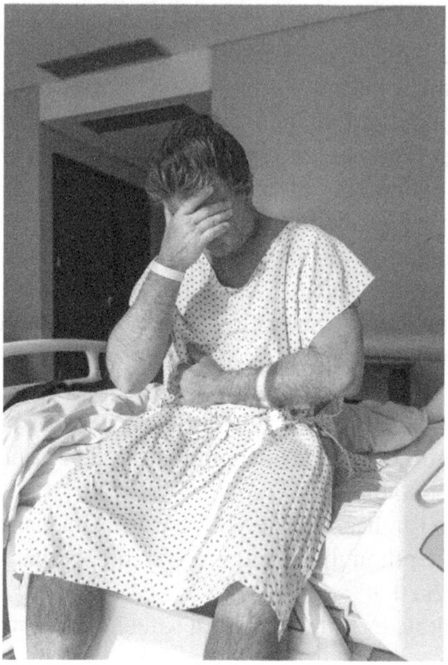

Figure 5.5 A patient gripping his abdomen in pain. Photo from Shutterstock.

morning while lifting boxes for his warehouse job. His EMR shows 12 ED visits over the past 18 months, all of which include similar pain-related complaints. All imaging contained in his chart suggests no structural abnormalities that could explain the source of his pain.

When speaking with the triage nurse, Nurse Cynthia West, Mr. Morales reports that over-the-counter medications offer little relief for his pain. He follows up with, "The only thing that ever works is what they give me here. I can't remember what it's called. It starts with a 'D'… 'Dah-something.'"

Providers: Nurse Cynthia West serves as the triage nurse on duty for the night-shift in the ED. She is the one to initially assess Mr. Morales' condition. His care is later managed by Dr. William Liu, an attending physician in the ED, and Dr. Samantha Stein, a first-year emergency medicine resident. Several other nurses, physician assistants, and medical students are also present as Mr. Morales' care gets transferred across providers.

Scenario: In this busy ED, clinicians are reviewing incoming patients on an electronic tracking board. One third-year medical student notes, "Ah, Morales is back at it." Another attending physician present responds, "Yep, earning his 'frequent flyer' miles," earning several head nods and chuckles from those at the workstation. Nurse West present continues the jest: "'Ten out of ten pain,' he says while scrolling his phone."

Upon entering the bay where Mr. Morales is waiting for further assessment, however, Nurse West's demeanor becomes much more serious. She introduces herself, establishes the patient's social history, and details his chief concern. She inquires about current and previous medications, during which time, Mr. Morales once again emphasizes that only the medications previously prescribed to him in the ED "ever even touch his pain." He states again, "I think it's called 'Dah-la' something."

"Dilaudid?" Nurse West asks.

"Yes! That's it. It's the only thing that helps."

Nurse West thanks Mr. Morales for his time, exits the bay, and pulls the curtain shut. She returns to the employee workstation, and says to Drs. Stein and Liu, "Morales always acts like he doesn't know exactly what he's asking for. He should have the word 'Dilaudid' ingrained in his mind by now." The exchange is overheard by a group of medical students, who seem to register the comment, but continue on with their work.

Dr. Liu then evaluates Mr. Morales. He explains that additional testing is necessary before stronger analgesics can be considered and so places orders for further imaging. Outside the bay and out of the patient's earshot, other clinicians recount Mr. Morales' history of frequent visits and the strategies they have employed to manage similar cases.

Later, when speaking to a group of medical interns, Dr. Stein refers to Mr. Morales using the same language she heard the other attending use early that evening, when he described the patient as a "frequent flyer."

Mr. Morales is prescribed 600 mg of ibuprofen every 6 hours for pain, but does not receive any opioid pain management. He is discharged with recommendations to follow up with his primary care physician.

Negotiating Professional Performances in the Front- and Backstages

The interactions featured here unfold across what the sociologist Erving Goffman (1959) terms the front- and backstages. Goffman employs the term "**frontstage**" to describe highly visible and highly performative areas of public life. By "performative," Goffman does not mean to imply that the actions undertaken in such spaces are disingenuous or otherwise feigned. Instead, he uses the term to signal how the interactions performed in such areas are highly scripted and guided by implicit institutional expectations that help to maintain the authority and perceived legitimacy of the professional role of "healthcare provider." Because the frontstage occurs in the view of others, all actions performed in such areas are subject to evaluation and individuals govern themselves accordingly. In the context of Case 3, the frontstage may be considered those areas in view of the patient. Nurse West and Dr. Liu operate in the frontstage (i.e., when interviewing and assessing Mr. Morales) in a way that is consistent with the professionalism expected of the role.

The **backstage** exists in contrast to the frontstage. In the context of the above case, the backstage is the workstation where various healthcare personnel congregate and converse about a variety of topics, but here, Mr. Morales in particular. Since the backstage is out of the public eye, it is where providers may express things deemed inappropriate or not socially acceptable for the frontstage. It is where they can communicate uncertainty, frustration, or in the case of Mr. Morales, skepticism—all of which would not be suitable to communicate in the frontstage. It is important to note, however, that the backstage does not represent a suspension of professionalism. The backstage serves a variety of functions: it is where clinicians coordinate patient care, where they "let off steam" related to the demands of the job, and where they forge intercollegial bonds. It is also where new members to the profession are socialized and how they are taught—albeit implicitly—how to interpret patient actions via a hidden curriculum.

Making the Hidden Curriculum Visible

The "**hidden curriculum**" refers to an informal mechanism of socializing members of a profession. The "hidden" part of this term therefore does not suggest subterfuge or intentional obfuscation. Instead, it signals that these learning experiences about what the medical profession entails and what it means to be a part of it are not transmitted through lectures and labs but through observations, off-the-cuff comments, and even disparaging jokes such as the one at the center of Case 3. We can see how the hidden curriculum being conveyed in backstage communication channels is at play here. An attending physician calls Mr. Morales a "frequent flyer"—a joking but pejorative term used to indicate that a patient often comes to the ED and presents with nebulous or difficult-to-verify symptoms. Dr. Stein overhears the other physician using this term and then later adopts it herself, demonstrating how the hidden curriculum is transmitted in subtle and frequently unintended ways.

Jokes like the one made at Mr. Morales's expense in Case 3 are a key feature of organizational culture. In her examinations of how healthcare providers negotiate their performances in both the front- and backstages, Ellingson (2009) shows how humor is positively used in the backstage by healthcare providers for the purposes of emotional regulation. After particularly taxing or emotionally draining patient encounters, Ellingson argues that oncology clinicians would use jokes to release emotional tension, create distance after intense empathetic encounters, and ultimately enable them to move on to the next patient. So, in this way, rather than undermine compassion as humor does in Case 3, in Ellingson's research, humor was used to sustain it.

To encourage providers to adopt helpful rather than hurtful varieties of humor, healthcare organizations may consider embedding humor awareness training into the new-employee onboarding curricula. Since humor serves multiple functions, outright suppression is both unrealistic and potentially disruptive to clinicians' workflows. Humor awareness training, however, could help providers distinguish between coping humor and categorizing humor. The former of these types of humor may help with regulating tension, whereas the latter often leads to patient stigmatization. Furthermore, in attempting to discern one type of humor from another, providers might ask themselves if they would be comfortable issuing such a joke in front of the patient. If not, then the joke may perhaps be left unsaid.

Admittedly, Ellingson (2009) also shows that patient categorization has its merits. Using this shorthand method for describing patients, for example, aids efficiency by distilling complex patient histories into recognizable organizational narratives. However, clinicians should be made aware of the highly consequential nature of patient categorization, as such labeling establishes the interpretative frame that providers will use even before meeting the patient. If the label were overtly negative (i.e., frequent flyer), it can color or distort the patient-provider interaction in a way that has profound health implications.

Two other interventions that healthcare organizations might adopt include making the hidden curriculum no longer hidden and modeling professionalism in the backstage. Studies have consistently shown the effects of the hidden curriculum become less pronounced when the hidden is made visible (Hafferty, 1998). The hidden curriculum may be made visible through processes of **metacommunication**, which is a commentary on the nature of communication itself. In practice, this might look like an attending asking a group of learners after rounds, "What assumptions might we have about this patient that are influencing our thinking here?" A simple reflexive question such as this takes implicit patient categorization and moves it into a place of conscious awareness.

That said, it would be difficult to dismantle the well-entrenched hidden curriculum of medicine overnight. So, what other mechanisms can be employed from within this hidden curriculum to create a more hospitable organizational culture for patients and providers alike? A primary way to change the hidden curriculum for the better is to leverage its in-built hierarchical systems. This would mean supervising healthcare personnel modeling professionalism, even in the backstage. So, if the "frequent flyer" remark introduced in Case 3 were to surface again, perhaps this time, the attending might say, "I suppose by that you mean that this patient is struggling with pain management. Let's see what we can do to help." Outside of these gentle pedagogical corrections, modeling behavior might also simply look like refraining from using such pejorative terms to describe patients—an easy feat for all members of the care team.

Speaking Up and Handing Off in Clinical Care

This chapter has demonstrated that communication in medicine happens interpersonally, but it also happens *organizationally*. Each individual interaction—between members of a care team or between a patient and a provider—is situated within a broader system of organizational norms, rituals, and culture.

Hierarchies, as a central feature of this culture, shape the direction that information travels, and even what constitutes relevant information. But it is key to understand that these hierarchies and communication channels are not contained within the organization; they make up the organization itself. If these channels change, so does the organization. This means that more equitable health organizations and more positive health outcomes are possible to produce by simply making different communicative choices.

Case 1 illustrates the communicative choices available to providers that may combat the detrimental effects of groupthink and preempt spirals of silence. It shows that what jeopardizes a patient's health is not simply poor clinical judgment or a misdiagnosis, but a climate wherein individuals do not feel safe to express dissent or voice uncertainty.

Case 2, however, homes in on handoffs to reframe communication not as the one-to-one transmission of information but a complex matter of translation and interpretation. When transferring care, clinicians are not only tasked with selecting which information is relevant and which is not, but also which is clinically actionable. The information that ends up being discarded is therefore not left out because the clinician does not notice it or take it into account, but because organizational norms privilege information that is easy to act upon. The proposed communication-based interventions for Case 2 (i.e., safety huddles and closed-loop communication) can thus be thought of as ways to help ensure that valuable information is being integrated into workflows all the same.

Finally, Case 3 spotlights the hidden curriculum. It draws upon Erving Goffman's dramaturgical metaphor of front- and backstages to better understand how members of the healthcare profession are socialized into it. The frontstage, as Case 3 shows, is where clinicians orient their communicative behaviors knowing that they are in full view of the patient. In the backstage, their interactions may be, at times, unprofessional (as illustrated by the "frequent flyer" joke), but this informal communication is how clinicians regulate emotions and engage in team building. The key, however, is to avoid certain kinds of backstage communication, such as labeling patients or otherwise categorizing them through humor, to prevent inadvertently supplying members of the care team with an interpretative frame that negatively impacts their ability to deliver impartial and compassionate care.

Yet, while each of these cases touches on a different communicative issue, they are all united in their implicit claim that changing health outcomes amounts to more than changing the ways individual healthcare workers communicate. It means changing the organizational culture in which they communicate—an organizational culture that determines what is said and under what circumstances, who gets to say it, and what, if anything, is done with that information. The following chapter, Chapter 6, adds another layer of complexity to these discussions of communication within organizations by considering how digital technologies likewise shape how information is stored, transmitted, and acted upon.

Glossary

- **Handoffs**
- **Organizational culture**
- **Groupthink**
- **Whistleblowers**
- **Sentinel event**
- **Closed-loop acknowledgment**
- **Frontstage**
- **Backstage**
- **Hidden curriculum**
- **Metacommunication**

Discussion Questions

1. Your attending says that a new case is coming that would offer you invaluable learning experiences and help make you more competitive for residency (or other career advancement opportunities). You are already nearing the 80-hour workweek cap, however. Working on this patient case would most certainly put you over that maximum limit. What would you do in this scenario?
2. If you saw an error committed on behalf of your attending/preceptor/charge nurse, but it did not have any bearing on patient health or well-being, would you report it? If so, how would you go about doing so?

Multimedia Resources

1. Learn more about closed-loop communication in clinical settings from the American Hospital Association: https://www.aha.org/center/project-firstline/teamstepps-video-toolkit
2. Listen to Dr. Danielle Ofri speak on the hidden curriculum of medicine and how it affects provider empathy: https://danielleofri.com/hidden-curriculum-of-medicine-video/

Further Reading

1. For further information on the history and present applications of groupthink, visit this summary presented by Ramon Aldag writing for the British Psychological Society: https://www.bps.org.uk/psychologist/groupthink-monument-truthiness
2. For an overview of the medical reforms initiated by the Libby Zion case, visit this New York Times article: https://www.nytimes.com/2009/03/03/health/03zion.html

References

Burke, L. G., Frakt, A. B., Khullar, D., Orav, E. J., & Jha, A. K. (2017). Association between teaching status and mortality in US hospitals. *JAMA, 317*(20), 2105–2113.

Dingley, C., Daugherty, K., Derieg, M. K., & Persing, R. (2008). *Improving patient safety through provider communication strategy enhancements.* In K. Henriksen, J. B. Battles, M. A. Keyes, & M. L. Grady (Eds.), *Advances in patient safety: New directions and alternative approaches* (Vol. 3, Performance and tools). Agency for Healthcare Research and Quality. https://www.ncbi.nlm.nih.gov/books/NBK43663/

Drolet, B. C., Schwede, M., Bishop, K. D., & Fischer, S. A. (2013). Compliance and falsification of duty hours: Reports from residents and program directors. *Journal of Graduate Medical Education, 5*(3), 368–373.

Eisenberg, E. M., Murphy, A. G., Sutcliffe, K., Wears, R., Schenkel, S., Perry, S., & Vanderhoef, M. (2005). Communication in emergency medicine: Implications for patient safety. *Communication Monographs, 72*(4), 390–413. https://doi.org/10.1080/03637750500322602

Ellingson, L. L. (2009). *Engaging crystallization in qualitative research: An introduction.* Sage.

European Parliament & Council of the European Union. (2003). *Directive 2003/88/EC of the European Parliament and of the Council of 4 November 2003 concerning certain aspects of the organisation of working time.* Official Journal of the European Union, L 299, 9–19. https://eur-lex.europa.eu/legal-content/EN/TXT/?uri=CELEX:32003L0088

Ghoul, I., Abdullah, A., Awwad, F., & Dardas, L. A. (2025). Safety huddle in healthcare settings: A concept analysis. *BMC Health Services Research, 25*(1), 393.

Goffman, E. (1959). *The presentation of self in everyday life.* Anchor Books.

Hafferty, F. W. (1998). Beyond curriculum reform: Confronting medicine's hidden curriculum. *Academic Medicine, 73*(4), 403–407.

Janis, I. L. (1972). *Victims of groupthink: A psychological study of foreign-policy decisions and fiascoes.* Houghton Mifflin.

Joint Commission. (n.d.). Sentinel events. https://www.jointcommission.org/resources/sentinel-event/

Kretchmar, J. (2021). *Groupthink.* EBSCO Research Starters. EBSCOhost.

Nasca, T. J., Day, S. H., & Amis, E. S. Jr. (2010). The new recommendations on duty hours from the ACGME Task Force. *New England Journal of Medicine, 363*(2), e3.

Noelle-Neumann, E. (1974). The spiral of silence a theory of public opinion. *Journal of Communication, 24*(2), 43–51.

Poulose, B. K., Ray, W. A., Arbogast, P. G., Needleman, J., Buerhaus, P. I., Griffin, M. R., & Holzman, M. D. (2005). Resident work hour limits and patient safety. *Annals of Surgery, 241*(6), 847–860.

Riesenberg, L. A. (2012). Shift-to-shift handoff research: Where do we go from here? *Journal of Graduate Medical Education, 4*(1), 4–8.

Salas, E., Wilson, K. A., Burke, C. S., & Wightman, D. C. (2006). Does crew resource management training work? An update, an extension, and some critical needs. *Human Factors, 48*(2), 392–412.

Sandroni, C., Nolan, J., Cavallaro, F., & Antonelli, M. (2007). In-hospital cardiac arrest: Incidence, prognosis and possible measures to improve survival. *Intensive Care Medicine, 33*(2), 237–245.

Schein, E. H. (1984). Coming to a new awareness of organizational culture. *Sloan Management Review, 25*(2), 3–16.

Williams, B. (2022). The national early warning score: From concept to NHS implementation. *Clinical Medicine, 22*(6), 499–505.

Williams, J. (2001). *Unbending gender: Why family and work conflict and what to do about it.* Oxford University Press.

6 Delivering Care in the Digital Age

The Medium Is the Message

For a long time, jokes about the illegibility of doctors' handwriting was a staple in medical culture, yet in today's healthcare landscape, such commentary is largely anachronistic. Indeed, handwritten patient charts, prescription requests, and specialist referrals are a thing of the past, as so much of healthcare communication has become digitized. It is perhaps the ubiquity of mediated communication—that is, communication that occurs through some channel or medium other than face-to-face—that implicitly encourages others to take its presence for granted. This chapter, however, aims for something different; it aims to reflect on how digital technologies actively shape communication in healthcare settings. Typically, these technologies are regarded as neutral instruments, a means to accomplish a particular end. Yet, here, we explore a different view. This chapter assumes that these channels of communication do not simply transmit information from one party to another—say, an oncologist nurse to an ICU attending—but fundamentally influences the message being conveyed. This perspective is in line with media theorist Marshall McLuhan's (1964) infamous declaration "The medium is the message." With this, McLuhan meant to suggest that the characteristics inherent within a particular medium (i.e., its speed, reach, and embeddedness within daily or organizational activities) carry just as much meaning as the content it "contains."

While McLuhan's insights were largely directed toward broadcast media such as television and radio, they are nonetheless applicable to the media that are routinely employed in clinical spaces. This chapter therefore begins by exploring arguably the most central digital medium within healthcare, the **electronic medical record (EMR)**, also referred to more colloquially by providers as "the patient chart." Case 1 interrogates how subtleties in the design and layout of that chart, as well as other documents used in these settings, influence communication dynamics. Included within this discussion is a consideration for the open-access quality of these systems, wherein patients can view directly their providers' clinical notes. This attention to open-access communication is

DOI: 10.4324/9781003654308-6

thus extended in Case 2, which examines how the abundance of medical information, which communication theorists frequently refer to as "information overload," available to patients via platforms like WebMD, social media, prominent health system websites, and even ChatGPT affects clinical communication. The "on-demand" nature of this information then sets the stage for Case 3, interrogating how the digital commercialization of healthcare in the way of direct-to-consumer platforms affects clinical communication by employing technology to shift medicine to a consumer-based model of care.

In order to impart this chapter conceptual balance, given that the cases presented above adopt a somewhat critical stance toward these technologies, the final case presented in this chapter, Case 3, serves to highlight the promise of such technologies. It explores how they can both improve providers' practice and serve equity initiatives by delivering care to those for whom it might otherwise be inaccessible. By concluding with this future-looking tone of possibility amidst an age of medicine thoroughly intertwined with new technologies, this chapter provides the ideal segue into the later conclusion of this book (Chapter 8), which essentially asks, "Where do we go from here?"

Case 1

Patient: Ms. Elena Kowalski, aged 57, is being admitted to the Hospital Universitario La Paz in Madrid for dyspnea and fatigue. Ms. Kowalski arrived at the hospital alone. Ms. Kowalski has recently immigrated to Spain from Poland. She moved here with her teenage children after divorcing her husband. Having no family around, she does not have consistent social or caregiving support. She works as a low-paid hotel maid and has to use public transportation to get to work while living in the outskirts of Madrid.

Scenario: Shortly upon arrival, Ms. Kowalski is handed a tablet to fill out intake forms, to be completed through the hospital's patient portal. She is prompted to answer a series of questions related to her employment status, occupation, the number of individuals living in her household, tobacco and alcohol use, primary language, and religious preferences. Several of these questions offer a space for short written responses, which she uses to note that her work as a housekeeper is irregular and thus often places significant financial strain on her and interferes with her ability to attend follow-up appointments.

Providers: Ms. Kowalski is being seen by Dr. Javier Morales, the internal medicine resident overseeing her admission, and Nurse Lucía Fernández, who administers Ms. Kowalski's intake.

As part of his charting duties, Dr. Morales must complete the Social History section of Ms. Kowalski's health record (Figure 6.1). When Dr. Morales opens the social history field in the patient's EMR, he encounters a dropdown menu consisting of boxes to check (e.g., employed v. unemployed, smoker v.

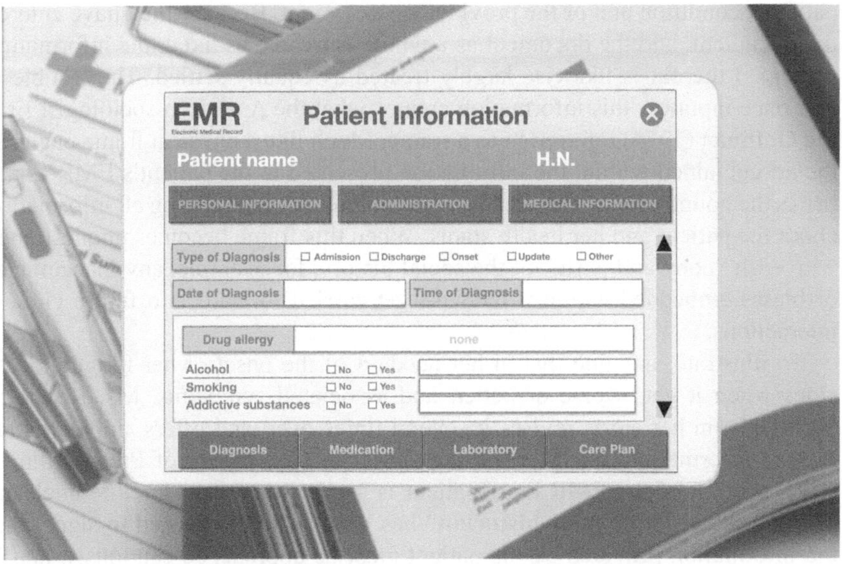

Figure 6.1 An example patient-viewing interface of an electronic medical record.

non-smoker, family history of cancer v. no history of such). At the bottom of the dropdown menu is a box for a short response, which allows enough space for the average text message (around 140 characters). Although Ms. Kowalski has provided additional contextual information regarding her unpredictable work schedule, her lack of social support, and her transportation as well as financial barriers, given the constraints of the system design, Dr. Morales simply writes, "Employed, lives with family, no tobacco, occasional alcohol, no family history of cancer."

Her issues are eventually resolved and she is discharged two days later. However, during subsequent follow-up visits with other clinics, the social history remains unchanged. Gradually, Ms. Kowalski's social circumstances become more unstable, but the entry in the social history box in her chart remains unchanged for several years. Multiple providers press the "skip this time" button in the medical record when reminded that the social history should be updated.

Far from "Neutral": Design, Language, and Authorship in EMRs

In medicine and public life in general, documents and texts are treated as largely static entities. In fact, it is only when something is put into writing that it is considered finalized. This is perhaps why many scholars have pointed out how difficult it is to contest diagnostic labels and loaded framing within the patient chart as they are "sticky"—that is, they remain in the chart despite changes in the patient's condition and/or the provider's assessment. Because they have entered the document, and the document as a whole is treated as fixed, the information presented therein is likewise largely treated as equally settled. The trouble is that once inputted, this information creates what the American sociologist Erving Goffman (1974) referred to as a frame. Much like a physical frame encloses the art contained within, the information presented in the patient's EMR establishes the boundaries, parameters, and guidelines for interpreting all information about the patient and her health status. When this frame becomes unquestioned with each "copy and paste" of the social history, for example, any inaccuracies or biases embedded within it likewise get carried forward into future clinical interactions.

To illustrate, imagine that in her account of the onset of her fatigue, occasions when it gets worse or better, and associated symptoms, Ms. Kowalski backtracks in her story, revises it several times over, and offers ample contradictory information. Dr. Morales thus notes in the History of Present Illness (HPI) portion of the EMR that "patient is a poor historian; timeline unclear." The use of the term "**poor historian**" has historically been used to signal that the information provided by the patient must be approached cautiously, and is not to be treated as purely factual or wholly accurate. This characterization of the patient as unreliable or untrustworthy, however, has been met with much criticism (see Vanka et al., 2025), especially because the use of the term is unevenly applied. In their analysis of over 13 million clinician notes spanning the time period from 2016 to 2023, Beach et al. (2025) used natural language processing to categorize the language providers employed to classify patients' credibility and competence. The researchers found that the notes included in their dataset were more likely to apply language undermining patient credibility (i.e., "poor historian") to Black patients than White ones. These findings have prompted the study authors to therefore suggest more neutral alternatives to "poor historian," which emphasize the extenuating circumstances that may prevent a patient from fully communicating details about their health; examples include "patient unable to provide a complete history" and "patient is uncertain about some details" (McCrear, 2025).

The results of Beach et al.'s (2025) study echo Chapter 3's premise that language affects perception, as the language providers employ in the EMR constructs the interpretative frame for all subsequent interactions with it. Once this frame is established, it becomes increasingly difficult to alter it, meaning that, in the case of the patients featured in Beach et al.'s (2025) study, existing biases and prejudices may only be further sedimented and compounded.

This phenomenon is what the academic literature on the subject refers to as "**diagnostic momentum**." In their article, "Seen through Their Eyes: Residents' Reflections on the Cognitive and Contextual Components of Diagnostic Errors in Medicine," Ogdie et al. (2012) define diagnostic momentum as "pushing forward diagnoses from previous encounters without evaluation of their accuracy or the goodness of fit with current presentation" (p. 1365). The authors cite handoffs (calling back to Chapter 5) as a primary site of this diagnostic momentum, wherein upon receiving a new patient under their care, providers often fail to question the information they receive about the patient or their diagnosis from the clinicians formerly overseeing their care. While previous chapters have interrogated handoffs as a juncture ripe for communication failures, the present one focuses on diagnostic momentum in the context of the patient EMR, specifically. One can appreciate the dangers of diagnostic momentum as it applies to Dr. Morales and Ms. Kowalski. If Dr. Morales were to label Ms. Kowalski a poor historian, this would supply the interpretative frame for all future providers interacting with her chart, perhaps coloring their interpretation of the information she provides. Ms. Kowalski's reporting of new or worsening symptoms, for example, may be dismissed since they are coming from a "poor historian," which could have a detrimental, and perhaps even deadly, effect on her overall health.

Indeed, once entered into the patient's EMR, information constitutes what Venkat (2015) refers to as "**chart lore**." For the author, chart lore occurs when information presented in the EMR is brought forward, often through repeated copying and pasting actions, but also through other providers who treat this provisional information that should ideally be subject to continuous review and revision as finalized and factual. Often, this is not done out of malice or even apathy; it occurs because of the institutional weight that documents carry. The weight granted to verbal contracts, oral promises, and other spoken expressions of commitment pale in comparison to those afforded to written ones precisely because of the fact that their individual authorship is obscured. Because documents like the EMR are the product of so many different authors, they, ironically, appear to be authored by no single person and thus inherently more objective—more of an accurate representation of reality (Goody, 1986; Latour, 1987). This perception, in turn, imbues clinical documents with staying power, as they recirculate within clinical spaces and across various communication channels among those who treat them as unquestionably authoritative. This chapter thus invites all clinicians to remain cognizant of the fact that these documents are composed by several individuals at various points in time, and as such, they remain tentative, open to amending, and inherently subjective.

This subjectivity may be further witnessed in the language providers adopt in the EMR. Even if Dr. Morales did not overtly label Ms. Kowalski a poor historian, there are other ways he may inadvertently characterize her as such. In the age of open-access EMRs, where patients can view the clinical summaries that providers write, providers are more aware of the word choices they make. Yet, this does not necessarily mean that they no longer express personal opinions or subjective appraisals. Amidst the constraints of open access, and acknowledging that patients will likely read what they write, providers may nonetheless convey their interpretations of the reliability of the patient's self-report in more nuanced linguistic terms.

Park et al. (2021), for instance, examine how something as simple as the reporting verbs used to convey information (e.g., patient *claims* and patient *believes*) can subtly influence how the recipient of such information may regard it. The authors note that "claims" and other "doubt markers" like "supposedly" and "apparently" function to signal the provider's skepticism concerning the information supplied by the patient. As the authors point out, even the way this information is presented can affect its interpretation. Quoted material is a case in point. Clinicians are taught to directly quote patients in their chart for reasons rooted in clinical accuracy and legal protections. What clinicians choose to quote, and how they introduce these quotes, is significant in terms of the patient picture they paint. Only quoting part of a statement, for example, may distort what the patient has said. Alternatively, the use of the quote marks themselves functions as scare quotes—as another way for clinicians to signal their skepticism over the veracity of the information a patient has provided (Park et al., 2021).

Self-Report, Questionnaires, and Diagnostic Likelihood

It is important to note, however, that communicating disbelief and uncertainty is not exclusively bad. In fact, as Chapter 5 demonstrated, expressing such uncertainty is a requisite of high-quality care. In communicating tentativeness or hesitation regarding the information presented in the EMR, one clinician is signaling to another that they may want to do further testing, engage the patient in another interview, or perform another physical exam to avoid diagnostic errors. As indicating uncertainty has been well-established in the literature as central to avoiding diagnostic error (Ilgen & Dhaliwal, 2025), there is utility to communicating such via the patient chart. A communication-based intervention in this regard, however, involves being transparent about this uncertainty. This would look like a move away from coded, implicit, and indirect language and toward less ambiguous alternatives. This might look like something as simple as writing "patient story unclear; recommend follow-up interview," which could convey uncertainty without undermining the patient's credibility.

Patient credibility is often further jeopardized when the only evidence a provider has to go off of is their self-report. Self-report, coupled with diagnostic questionnaires (see Figure 6.2), are some of the primary means of measuring conditions that cannot be verified through empirical means such as labwork, imaging, and physical exam. Key examples include psychiatric disorders and learning disabilities. In both cases, the provider cannot readily observe the condition and can therefore not verify its existence in a manner consistent with the positivist orientation that is so pervasive in medicine and the sciences (refer to Chapter 1). To legitimize these conditions in the absence of physical signs, clinicians employ instruments like diagnostic questionnaires. Yet, much like the patient's EMR, these documents are likewise by no means neutral.

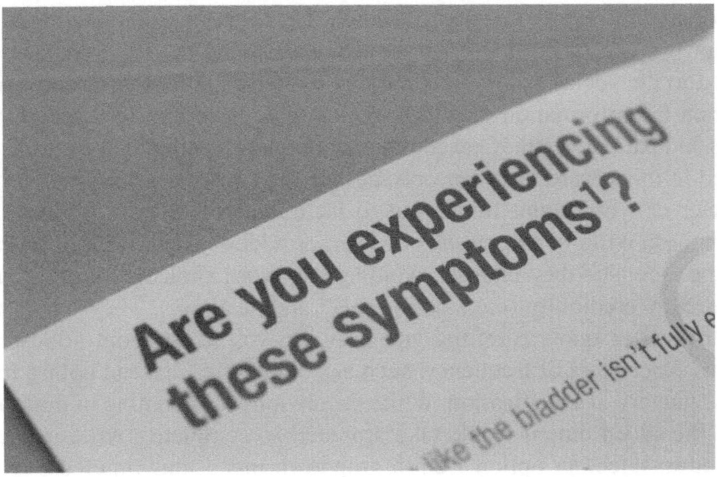

Figure 6.2 An example diagnostic questionnaire. Photo from Shutterstock.

Typically, these questionnaires assume the form of a series of statements that the patient agrees or disagrees with to varying degrees of frequency and intensity. These Likert-type based assessments will thus present the patient with a statement like, "I have little interest in doing things" and then offer them options for responding, such as "Most of the time," "Often," "Sometimes," "Rarely," and "Never." Common examples of such questionnaires include the well-known Beck Depression Inventory (BDI) and the Patient Health Questionnaire-9 (PHQ-9). Forbes (2015), however, shows how these documents do much more than simply collect information; their very design determines how this information is interpreted and acted upon. In her analysis of an ADHD diagnostic questionnaire used by an outpatient psychiatric office, the author shows how the spatial layout of the document itself guides the patient toward a preferred response. The columns for indicating the frequency with which a patient experiences a particular symptom are presented in varying degrees in width. High frequencies like "Frequently" and "Very Frequently" are granted much more physical space than "Rarely" and "Never." In fact, the column for "Never" is so narrow that it has to be written vertically. By physically making it difficult to check this box through a narrowed column, the document discourages the patient from this response. What this ultimately translates to is more patients checking boxes denoting higher symptom frequency, and thus a greater number of individuals receiving an ADHD diagnosis. Therefore, as Forbes shows, the design of these documents can subtly privilege certain responses, which, in turn, influences diagnostic outcomes.

While the document that Forbes (2015) analyzes was a physical paper-based one, the insights garnered are nonetheless applicable to a digital context.

Referring to the type of digital document Dr. Morales in interacting with, the dropdown menu of pre-loaded response options and the brief character count allotted to the social history section may likewise guide, shape, and otherwise constrain the information provided, which may, in turn, affect diagnostic outcomes and patient health. One communication intervention that could be implemented in this regard is to not only design short response sections with larger character or word count limits, but to include more write-in options overall. Within these write-in responses, however, providers would want to be cautious with the language they choose, avoiding any word choice that might question the patient's credibility (e.g., "seemingly" and "claims"). They would also be well-advised to quote carefully and fully, as well as to avoid hollow or ambiguous descriptors of frequency, such as "frequently," instead opting for more precise numerical specification. While the obvious shortcoming of this approach lies in the added time it would take providers to complete a write-in section as opposed to select an option from a dropdown menu, this time cost is usually measurable in seconds and provides benefits to patient health that far outweigh the risks associated with a narrowly designed diagnostic tool.

Another actionable intervention targets the practice of copying and pasting previously written social histories. To dissuade clinicians from doing this, they might double-check the accuracy of the social history during visits, just as one would a medication list. Inquiring about new or changed medications at the beginning of a patient visit is standard practice across specialities. Therefore, it would be relatively easy to build upon this line of questioning by adding one dedicated to ensuring the up-to-date status and accuracy of the social history.

While Case 1 has demonstrated the significance of the patient chart in shaping health outcomes, and how they may even exacerbate existing health inequities, the truth is that they are just one of many digital platforms that individuals engage with. From the phones in most people's pockets to the laptops and tablets they use for work, to the commercials that interrupt the movie they are streaming, the average person is presented with an abundance of mediated information. It is therefore not surprising that some of this input would show up in the healthcare interaction. Case 2 moves beyond the EMR, considering the impact of other digital mechanisms patients interface with every day upon the healthcare they receive.

Case 2

Patient: Ms. Jill Taylor is a 32-year-old, otherwise healthy, female who presents with concerns about weight gain and fatigue. She self-scheduled online with an endocrinologist, Dr. Paek. This visit takes place in an outpatient clinic in a suburb of Phoenix, Arizona (U.S.). The practice has recently introduced online self-scheduling to compete with other local hospitals and practices by improving patient access to providers and to cut down on the number of staff needed for phone scheduling.

Scenario: Ms. Taylor is a defense lawyer and has gained about 20 pounds in the past year. She has had regular gynecologic check-ups over the years to have her birth control refilled and recently discontinued use of oral contraceptives in favor of an IUD. She made her appointment with Dr. Paek after seeing a social media video of someone with similar symptoms who was diagnosed with hypothyroidism. Her gynecologist ordered a "TSH with reflex to T4" last week, which resulted in a normal TSH, so no T4 testing was performed.

Provider: Dr. Paek is an endocrinologist who has been in practice for 32 years. He has practiced at several teaching hospitals but joined his current multispecialty practice when he and his wife moved to be closer to their adult children. He is planning to retire next year.

Dr. Paek begins the visit by discussing Ms. Taylor's symptoms. She endorsed the above weight gain and stated that she frequently felt tired, though this could be due to frequent nighttime anxiety about her work. She denied constipation and cold intolerance but does have some occasional dry skin, usually in cold weather. Her menstrual cycles did not change until she stopped her oral contraceptives. Dr. Paek performs a thorough physical exam, including a thyroid exam, which is normal. He tells Ms. Taylor that he does not think a thyroid problem would explain her symptoms, in light of the normal TSH. He did not recommend repeat testing.

Visibly frustrated, Ms. Taylor mentions that her social media feed had presented her with ads for direct-to-consumer healthcare platforms that advertise quick diagnosing and medication for thyroid disorders, weight gain, and fatigue mailed directly to her door. She expresses a sense of frustration that she feels her providers are "gatekeeping" these resources from her, especially when they are available through a few "clicks of a button (Figure 6.3)." Ms. Taylor insists

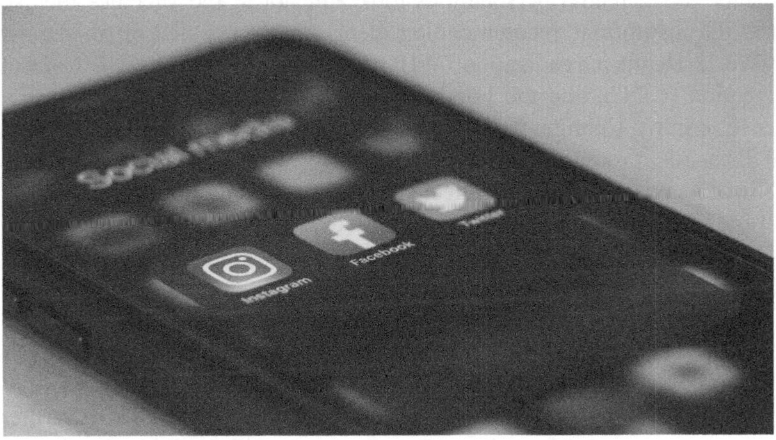

Figure 6.3 A phone with social media icons. Photo from Shutterstock.

that she wants to have repeat TSH testing done, also with a free T4, T3, thyroglobulin antibodies, and TPO antibodies. The social media personality from her video said these were necessary to diagnose the thyroid problem. Ms. Taylor also asked an online AI chatbot whether hypothyroidism could be missed with just a TSH, and it said that it could.

Patient Autonomy and Provider Authority

Throughout much of modern history, medicine has been a well-entrenched social authority. As discussed in Chapter 1, such social authority is reflected in how, up until very recently, if one needed to miss school or work, they would be tasked with securing a "doctor's note" excusing them from their duties. And even today, if one is requesting disability benefits from the government, worker's compensation for an on-the-job injury, or a permit for handicapped parking, a healthcare provider must formally attest to and vouch for the patient's need for such things. The fact that providers are put in a position to testify in such a way, in turn, solidifies their status as a social authority and their ability to adjudicate over several areas of life, not just the ones that are exclusively medical. But now, medicine must contend with new social authorities in the form of digital media and artificial intelligence (AI). The threats that digital (particularly, social) media and AI pose to patient health hardly need restating. With respect to social media, specifically, the anti-vaccine (i.e., "anti-vaxx") movement that flourished on social media during and after the COVID-19 pandemic is an illustrative case in point. Social media personalities with followings in the millions made baseless claims asserting that SARS-CoV-2 vaccines caused female infertility, for instance. Such claims translated to action, as Wang et al. (2022) note, as more couples undergoing artificial insemination fertility treatments declined the vaccine.

Other social media personalities took aim not at the vaccines themselves, but at the institutions recommending them. Long-esteemed organizations like the World Health Organization (WHO), the Centers for Disease Control and Prevention (CDC), and the Food & Drug Administration (FDA) came under intense scrutiny. Changes to these agencies' respective recommendations for social distancing protocols and vaccine schedules were interpreted by much of the public as inconsistencies that reflected duplicitous or ulterior motives rather than simply the institutions responding to new evidence as it was received (Pollard & Davis, 2022). In this vacuum of social authority that was thus created, a new social authority stepped in.

For many, parasocial relationships came to fill the void that medicine—as represented by these key institutions—left behind. "Parasocial relationships," as Kim et al. (2024) define them, "refer to the imaginary human relationships formed between media audiences and media figures" (p. 282). Often, the relationships online users form in such contexts are with individuals who possess little to no health expertise or credentialing. In fact, it is their appearance as an average citizen "just like me" that makes these figures both relatable and appealing to many. However, the very notion of "authority" has come to be reconstituted in the online realm. Many healthcare providers have assumed a new hybrid role of practitioner-influencer. And while some of these providers leverage the visibility of their platform in the interest of public health, by correcting circulating misinformation, for example, others use it to market products or services they are compensated to endorse. This dual role that many providers inhabit thus invites questions as to the ethics of this practice as well as the scope of their professional boundaries—a subject to be discussed at greater length in Case 3. To return to Ms. Taylor, however, her references to social media can thus be interpreted simply as a continuation of this trend. Dr. Paek may choose to respond, as many providers do, by expressing contempt for such online sources, or even disdain for the fact that these influencers' recommendations are being placed on par with his own. Or, in a more productive manner, he may seek to understand how these resources function for Ms. Taylor.

As previously established in Chapter 1, the social authority conveyed to medicine has also given rise to paternalism, wherein medicine and its representatives are positioned as knowing what is best for the patient. In many ways, Ms. Taylor's actions (consulting social media and AI) may be interpreted as a reaction against such paternalism. Such resources may allow patients to feel as though they are decentralizing power once exclusively held with the provider, enacting their own autonomy, and engaging in the shared decision-making that is championed by medicine. Admittedly, there are many patients for whom such an approach lacks appeal. For them, they arrive at the healthcare interaction seeking expertise—to essentially be told what to do (see Caronia in Bartesaghi and Forbes (2026) for further elaboration on this critique of shared decision-making). As they see it, one does not take their car to a mechanic to be asked what they think the problem is, so the same applies to their own health. Yet, there are still patients like Ms. Taylor who do want to weigh in on their own health matters, and use peer and digital resources to do so.

So, what should Dr. Paek do in this situation? Surely, he cannot ignore the evidence in the form of lab results before him. But to indulge Ms. Taylor's request for additional testing without sufficient grounds it would also constitute a lack a responsible medical **resource stewardship**[1] and give credence to a misguided model of medicine rooted in perpetually expanding diagnostic testing rather than clinical reasoning. What he can do instead is to review the lab results in a transparent manner, explaining why further testing is unlikely to yield greater insights. Instead of simply refusing to pursue further testing, which would be an exercise in paternalism, he should explain that this line of diagnostic inquiry may serve as a red herring, directing attention where it is not warranted and thus obscuring investigation into more worthy areas. By emphasizing how further testing can therefore work against Ms. Taylor's wishes for her health—that is, addressing the weight gain, fatigue, and so on—and underscoring that these goals are mutual, he validates rather than discredits her commitment to finding an answer. He moreover does this not by denigrating the sources she has based her decisions on, but by returning to the body of evidence before him.

Social media has also introduced Ms. Taylor to direct-to-consumer healthcare platforms, such Hims/Hers, Nurx, and Fridays. Platforms such as these adopt a common business model, which typically involves a patient inputting limited healthcare data on a screening form. This information is then sent to a remote provider for review. Then, often without even speaking to the patient, the provider sends in a prescription, which is mailed to the patient's door. As is apparent in Ms. Taylor's comments about gatekeeping, the ease with which patients can access medications through such services has reshaped medicine today by shifting it more to a consumer model. Patients are no longer patients, per se; they are customers. And providers are now tasked with providing exceptional customer service in the guise of bedside manner. This consumer model of medicine is also evident in online review systems like Google Review, through which a patient can rate a provider or practice just as they would a pizza parlor. The commercialization of medicine, as represented by review systems and direct-to-consumer healthcare platforms, forces providers to navigate several competing tensions. For one, they must practice evidence-based medicine, but they must also find ways that ensure that the patient leaves the interaction feeling satisfied.

In Case 1, Dr. Paek adheres to the tenets of evidence-based medicine by restating, summarizing, and interpreting Ms. Taylor's test results, and how they do not suggest further testing should be done. But doing so appears to only frustrate Ms. Taylor further, as she "insists" on repeat testing. The question then becomes one of how to balance these competing demands. What Dr. Paek could do is acknowledge the presence of these new players in the field of medicine and articulate to Ms. Taylor how they differ from the practice of medicine traditionally conceived. He may emphasize that the diagnostic efficiency and scale at which these platforms operate are oriented toward customer satisfaction and not necessarily clinical accuracy. Instead of moralizing such platforms, however, by positioning these platforms as lesser than conventional medical models, he may highlight the tradeoffs inherent within them. Dr. Paek may, for example, underscore that these platforms work well when there are clear diagnostic indicators (e.g., a patient has already received a diagnosis and now just wants access to medication). However, if a patient's diagnosis is unclear, as in Ms. Taylor's case, Dr. Paek could stress the importance of traditional clinical care, which is designed for longitudinal assessment and better suited for risk management.

AI, Bias, and Clinical Decision-Making

But Ms. Taylor's request for additional testing is only partially informed by social media. She also fed her symptoms into AI software that confirmed that hypothyroidism could be missed if just going off of TSH values alone (Figure 6.4). While the use of AI for diagnostic purposes is relatively new, AI itself is not. In fact, the term "artificial intelligence" has been around since the 1950s (McCarthy et al., 2006) and used to refer to anything from the software used to filter and select flights for a vacation to the fraud-detection one has embedded into their credit card and banking systems. Humanity has long been using AI to guide decision-making processes. For example, AI-based credit score systems play an integral role in approving mortgage loans; they routinely influence recommendations for news story delivery; screen resumes to determine which job applicants will be shortlisted for an interview; and even calculate insurance plan premiums. The difference is that while before, these systems were only available to smaller groups of individuals, now, many of them—the system that Ms. Taylor used included—are open-access. The changes in access to AI systems therefore invites questions regarding its responsible and ethical use. Is Ms. Taylor's consulting AI any different than a physician watching a YouTube video of a procedure they have not performed in a while prior to doing that procedure in real life? In both cases, the individual turning to AI resources is utilizing the system to learn from their peers—to have all of the information on the internet searched, filtered, and then packaged in a meaningful way.

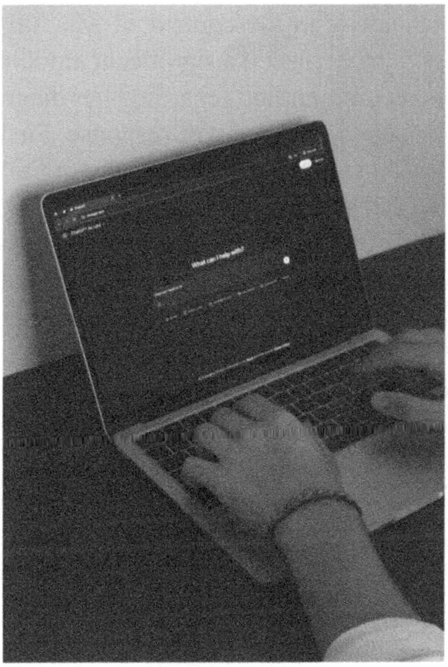

Figure 6.4 A person interacting with a generative AI platform. Photo from Unsplash.

The problem enters when one acknowledges that AI systems, just like the digital EMR, are not neutral tools. AI systems are often talked about in the same breath as machine learning, precisely because many AI platforms are designed to learn—to provide more tailored or informed recommendations—with greater feedback and input from users. However, when such systems are not presented with a comprehensive dataset to learn from, their outputs are equally skewed and often biased. In an article examining the use of AI-informed treatment recommendations for lung cancer, Ding et al. (2024)[2] found the model's performance varied across patient subgroups. More specifically, the model exhibited lower accuracy in predicting appropriate treatment categories for patients under 60 when compared to patient groups 60 and older. Its recommendations also faltered along the lines of disease type, with the recommendation classifications for adenocarcinoma proving less accurate than squamous cell carcinoma, even though adenocarcinoma has a higher incidence rate among the general population. These discrepancies in performance may be explained by the composition of the dataset on which the AI model was trained. The model was trained on an imbalanced, synthetic dataset, one that included few cases of adenocarcinoma presentations among younger patients. As a result, the model overrepresented certain patient groups in its recommendations.

What this example shows is that when AI systems are trained on incomplete or otherwise biased data, they tend to perpetuate such biases in a way that has direct implications for patient health. In this case, an improperly trained AI model may offer recommendations that benefit some patients while quietly excluding others. This is an important takeaway in the context of Ms. Taylor's case, considering that Ms. Taylor appears to have placed a significant amount of faith in what the AI system she consulted is recommending regarding her diagnosis. In the above case, Dr. Paek may wish to engage in a three-part response. First, he is advised to resist interpreting the patient's AI consultations as an attempt to discredit or undermine his expertise. In seeking out AI assistance, Ms. Taylor is simply engaged in what Weick (1995) refers to as "sensemaking," wherein individuals aim to interpret uncertain or ambiguous situations by retrospectively organizing their experiences into a cogent narrative. This is precisely what Ms. Taylor is doing here—she is attempting to make sense of her symptoms in seeking a diagnosis. The power of sensemaking as a motivator for behavior is evidenced by the fact that patients often feel relief in receiving a diagnosis, even if there is no treatment plan or therapeutic intervention available for it (Sims et al., 2021). Ms. Taylor is therefore also likely to be looking for relief—not just relief from her symptoms, which may or may not be possible, but relief from the perpetual uncertainty over what is going on in her body. Recognizing this will encourage any provider, Dr. Paek included, to interpret her AI and social media consultations in a more empathetic light—as simply a desire to make sense of what is happening to her.

The second part of the three-part response Dr. Paek may wish to adopt involves validating her desire to become an active participant in her own healthcare. While taking care to not come across as patronizing, Dr. Paek can commend Ms. Taylor on the proactive behavior she has taken with respect to her own health. Doing this acknowledges Ms. Taylor's desire to exercise autonomy with respect to her health. He may even go so far as to cite evidence speaking to the fact that patients typically witness better outcomes when they are active participants in their own care (Hibbard & Greene, 2013).

The final part of Dr. Paek's response, however, is perhaps the most important. He must be careful to acknowledge the limitations of AI. First among these is that AI deals in possibilities, not probabilities; it introduces outcomes that are possible, regardless of their likelihood to occur in an actual clinical context. Clinical reasoning rooted in experience and contextual cues, however, does the exact opposite. Clinical reasoning is also informed by physical exam findings (or the lack thereof), interactional nuances derived from the patient interview, and years of experience practicing medicine. Finally, just like humans, AI is not impartial, despite giving the appearance that it is. While AI systems may not have a vested interest in diagnostic outcomes, when making recommendations based on incomplete or biased data, it may be equally subject to one-sided interpretation. Dr. Paek may therefore frame it as a valuable resource for Ms. Taylor, but one that should also be supplemental, auxiliary, or secondary to clinical judgment.

Admittedly, the picture painted thus far of AI technologies in healthcare has adopted a largely pessimistic portrayal. Case 3, however, attempts to offer a more balanced view by considering not only the potential pitfalls of AI, but its promise as well.

Case 3

Patient: Mr. Wheeler is a 67-year-old male with a history of hypertension and Type 2 diabetes. He lives in a rural part of Missouri, in the American Midwest, about two hours from the nearest medical center.

Scenario: Mr. Wheeler meets with Dr. Lawson via video conferencing. Through the telehealth platform, Dr. Lawson performs a standard medical history intake and visual assessment. He is seeing Dr. Lawson, a physician at his primary care clinic, via telehealth for a "sick" visit (Figure 6.5). He reports intermittent shortness of breath and swelling of his lower extremities. Mr. Wheeler has a history of not being able to attend his follow-up appointments due to transportation issues.

Provider: Trained in family medicine, Dr. Lawson is one of five doctors practicing in a clinic serving a rural area with a dispersed patient population. Much like her colleagues, she has a large patient panel, seeing, on average, 25–30 patients a day. She does not have a medical assistant or scribe on her team, so she carries a heavy administrative burden with respect to documentation, coordinating care, and scheduling. To ease this burden, her clinic has recently introduced AI-assistive technologies in the form of scribing tools and decision-guided prompts within the electronic medical record.

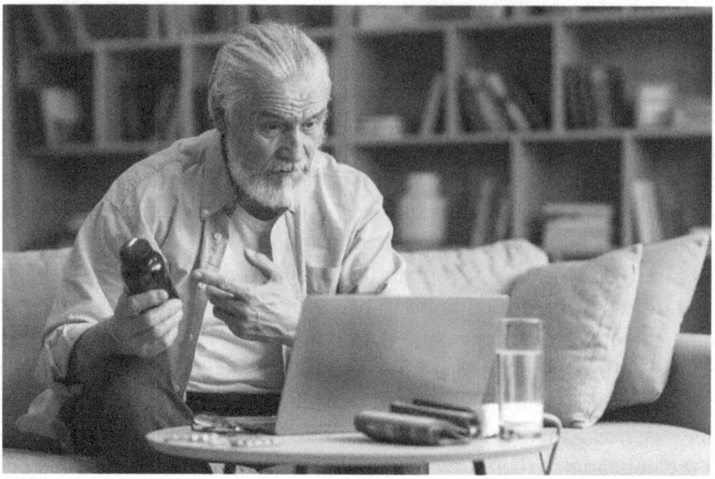

Figure 6.5 An elderly patient engaged in a telehealth visit.

While interviewing Mr. Wheeler, she does not type on her computer or take other notes, instead allowing the AI scribe to do this for her. As she is talking through Mr. Wheeler's symptoms, she hears a "ping" coming from her workstation computer. It is an AI alert suggesting that, given Mr. Wheeler's combination of symptoms, vitals, and medical history, she should consider early congestive heart failure as a diagnosis.

Alert Fatigue: Too Much of a Good Thing?

Consistent with clinical trends in the present day, AI appears at several junctures in Dr. Lawson's practice. The first place it appears is as a diagnostic verification tool embedded within Mr. Wheeler's EMR. AI for decision support purposes is being rolled out in a variety of healthcare contexts. One such example is the Epic Sepsis Model, an AI clinical decision support (CDS) tool embedded in the well-known EMR management system, EPIC, generates risk scores and alerts for sepsis, thus flagging patients in need of further evaluation (Wong et al., 2021). Johns Hopkins University recently developed a similar early warning notification system that continuously analyzes information in the patient's EMR and alerts providers for possible risks. This system, referred to as TREWS (Targeted Real-Time Early Warning System), shows great promise, as Adams et al. (2022) found that the model's performance among nearly 600,000 patients across five hospitals resulted in significantly lower mortality rates if the clinician responded to the TREWS alert within three hours.

This study's findings that the AI model's ability to reduce patient mortality rates is contingent upon the provider's timely response to the alert is an important point worth further consideration. Providers may adopt a variety of responses to these alerts, but one of most significant obstacles these models have to overcome pertains to the concept of alert fatigue. Well-established within the academic literature, alert fatigue refers to a phenomenon in which providers receive so many alerts and notifications that they become desensitized to them, leading to them ultimately ignoring or overriding these alerts. For instance, studies have shown that as a result of alarm fatigue, providers overrode automated drug-to-drug interaction alerts more than 90% of the time (Bryant et al., 2014). So, the likelihood that Dr. Lawson will act upon the AI alert she receives when examining Mr. Wheeler may depend on how many alerts she has already received throughout the day (i.e., her alert fatigue).

Fatigue may also enter in the context of provider fatigue. Providers with a heavy workload or those experiencing burnout may be at risk of overrelying on AI alerts to guide their decision-making. Decision-making is a cognitively taxing process, and especially in settings like the one in which Dr. Lawson finds herself, where providers must contend with a particularly high patient volume, it may be tempting to offload decision-making to AI entirely. Additionally, while there are those who may favor AI for the time-saving measures it offers, there are a fair number of providers who are skeptical of AI. Their bias therefore lies at the other end of the spectrum from those who may blindly follow its decisional guidance. As Tun et al. (2025) note, reasons for this bias may stem from the lack of transparency inherent in AI decision-making processes, changes to the provider-patient relationship, and an overreliance or dependency on these tools. What clinicians like Dr. Lawson must therefore bear in mind is that AI in healthcare operates in a complex organizational system, one that is vulnerable to complications stemming from both provider fatigue and human bias. Overreliance on automation should be cautioned against, as AI is best implemented as a supplement—not a substitute—for human decision-making. At the same time, however, in light of the above-referenced evidence supporting AI's ability to lower mortality rates and improve health outcomes, its integration into clinician workflows appears warranted. It is up to providers, though, to ensure this integration remains ethical, responsible, and sustainable.

The Associated Costs of AI

Within this episode, in addition to CDS, AI also appears as an auxiliary scribe. It is at this point, however, that critics may raise concerns about staff replacement—an often-invoked narrative surrounding AI for use in the workplace. Certainly, these claims are not unfounded, as several multinational organizations like Amazon and Google have cited AI as the reason for large-scale employee layoffs (Cunningham, 2026). Within healthcare, however, AI for scribing purposes may actually prevent employee attrition. As a speciality, family medicine is highly susceptible to provider turnover, as are other primary care specialties, including OB/GYN (Willard-Grace et al., 2019). One well-documented reason behind this attrition is the burnout brought on by extensive administrative duties. On the topic of provider burnout, Underdahl et al. (2024) write, "Long working hours, high patient volumes, administrative tasks, and limited control over work schedules amplify stress levels among physicians." The authors continue that EHRs, which were originally introduced to ease the administrative burden placed on providers, have ironically increased it by creating increased documentation demands. These claims are supported by survey data from Kane (2020), which found that nearly 50% of physicians across 29 specialties reported experiencing burnout. In a report of the study's findings, Dr. Frank John Ninivaggi of Yale New Haven Hospital noted, "The number of physicians feeling burned out is fairly consistent. The leading cause is administrative burden, as driven by workplace and organizational culture."

The burden brought on by the increased need for documentation presents a unique opportunity to offload certain tasks to AI. Scribing is just one of the tasks that AI can perform. As Case 3 demonstrates, Dr. Lawson's use of AI scribing tools allows her to signal that Mr. Wheeler has her full attention. By freeing up her hands from having to type while Mr. Wheeler is speaking, and by preventing her from having to face a computer screen, the AI scribing tools Dr. Lawson employs allow her to avoid many of the traditional pitfalls of nonverbal communication described in Chapter 4. With the use of these scribing tools, which run in the background, capturing key details of the conversation, Dr. Lawson can maintain eye contact, she can engage in minimal responses that suggest she is paying attention (e.g., head nodding and the like), and perhaps even more importantly, attend to any nonverbal cues displayed by Mr. Wheeler suggesting that alternative lines of inquiry should be pursued. Indeed, the ability of AI to free up clinician's time to focus on the patient is why the majority of 2,000 patients featured in a survey said they would be in favor of AI in clinical encounters provided that patient consent was secured (Leiserowitz et al., 2025).

Greater patient satisfaction, in turn, often leads to increased institutional revenue. This holds important implications for a practice such as Dr. Lawson's, which is both independent and operating in a rural area. In the U.S., where Dr. Lawson's clinic is operating, healthcare systems are run on a **fee-for-service financial model**, meaning that rather than being paid a flat fee, providers are paid for each individual procedure they perform, test they order, and exam they administer. The fees one can assess furthermore vary based on the complexity of the physician's task. This is a primary feature of the U.S. healthcare system, one that distinguishes it from its Canadian, European, and U.K. counterparts. Further distinguishing the U.S. from other similarly developed nations is the fact that healthcare in the U.S. is rooted in a **multi-payer system**, wherein payment is derived from multiple sources, including private insurers, government-sponsored programs like Medicare and Medicaid, and patient self-pay. This is in direct contrast to the **single-payer system** adopted by many other countries, where the government, as represented by the National Health Service (NHS) in the U.K., for example, funds patient care.

The financial constraints imposed by the system in which Dr. Lawson practices thus deliver additional challenges to remaining financially solvent. Unlike urban centers, rural clinics often serve fewer patients, and fewer patients means fewer services to bill for. That said, Case 3 notes that Dr. Lawson has a high patient volume, seeing approximately 25–30 patients a day. However, in this setting, more patients may not always translate to more revenue for the clinic. Many patients in rural areas such as the one in which Dr. Lawson is practicing are **underinsured** (Georgetown University Health Policy Institute, n.d.). This does not mean that the patient is *uninsured*, necessarily, but that they have high out-of-pocket costs or their insurance **deductible** (the amount the patient must first pay before their insurance will issue reimbursement) is high relative to their annual income (Commonwealth Fund, 2024). Because uninsured patients means care goes uncompensated and government-backed programs like Medicaid reimburse providers at lower rates than private insurers, clinics with this payer mix typically receive less revenue per visit. The clinics are then tasked with offsetting these costs by increased patient volume, as in Dr. Lawson's case.

Over time, however, issues with reimbursement can place independent clinics like this at risk, making them a prime target for acquisition by larger hospital systems. Within the U.S., multi-state hospital systems like HCA Healthcare, Kaiser Permanente, and Trinity Healthcare, to name a few, are becoming more common and slowly edging out local independent clinics within the healthcare marketplace. When under financial strain, clinics like Dr. Lawson's lack bargaining power and are more likely to be acquired by such hospital systems. Once this transfer of ownership happens, standardization protocols that limit provider autonomy often follow, as do a narrowing of services offered. So, while acquisition may protect clinics from falling financially asunder in the short-term, in the long-term, this consolidation may exert a negative impact on patient care.

AI is uniquely poised to address such concerns by reducing staffing needs, which translates to reduced downstream costs. While on the one hand, using AI for such purposes plays into existing fears about such technologies replacing human labor forces, on the other hand, its implementation may be viewed less as a substitute and more as a redistribution of labor. By freeing up providers' time spent on administrative tasks, AI can allow them to focus on other tasks with greater impact. For instance, Chapter 1's discussion of narrative medicine notes that the practice has appealing theoretical roots and ideological commitments but fails to adequately translate to practical contexts, in large part due to institutional incentives that encourage providers to see as many patients as possible in the least amount of time (due to the fee-for-service model aforementioned).

Relative value units (RVUs) are a central feature of American healthcare. Set by the Center for Medicare and Medicaid Services (CMS), each procedure that can be performed by a physician is assigned a set amount of RVUs based on its perceived complexity, the liability involved, overhead costs and so on. For many institutions, provider compensation is determined, at least in part, by RVUs generated by that individual provider. A possible advantage of integrating

AI into medical care would be to allow more patients to be seen, and thus possibly more procedures or care to be delivered; this, in turn, increases an individual provider's productivity. This would have the knock-on effect of increasing their compensation, assuming the current compensation model stayed stable. In theory, if an AI could write a provider's notes, for example, it could also allow more time for narrative medicine to be used when seeing patients.

The final benefit that AI tools may deliver, as illustrated by Case 3, is its ability to overcome the barriers imposed by distance. As the case notes, Mr. Wheeler's lack of access to reliable transportation makes receiving follow-up care difficult, and his experiences are representative of those of countless other patients. For example, in their comparative analysis of the barriers faced by parents of children with special needs in accessing healthcare in urban and rural areas, Skinner and Slifkin (2007) identified transportation to be a key hindrance to accessing care separating rural residents from their urban counterparts. Telehealth visits powered by AI technologies, however, can help overcome the limitations of geographic location. This, in turn, translates to improved health outcomes for patients in rural areas, who typically exhibit worse health outcomes across multiple domains, including general mortality, cardiac-related mortality, stroke-related mortality, and unintentional injury mortality (Cross & Warraich, 2021).

The potential of AI to surmount geographical divides extends well beyond a U.S., or even a Western context. Researchers have developed AI software that could guide healthcare workers in sub-Saharan Africa to capture high-quality fetal ultrasound images for diagnostic purposes (Gomes et al., 2022). The AI system uses real-time feedback on where to place the transducer to obtain biometric measurements. In cases such as these, the AI system is not intended to replace qualified obstetricians, but rather to deliver prenatal care to populations that would otherwise remain unserved.

In addition to geographic equity, AI for use in healthcare delivery may also address socioeconomic disparities. For many, middle-of-the-day clinic visits mean missed work, and missed work means missed income. When more than half (57%) of the world's workforce is living paycheck to paycheck, missing work to attend a health visit may be unfeasible (ADP, 2025). However, the emergence of telehealth may allow patients to meet with a provider during their lunch break or afterhours. As people living paycheck to paycheck experience greater health disparities due to the barriers imposed by their socioeconomic status, AI is therefore poised to overcome these barriers to improve health outcomes.

Digital Technologies in Health: Its Promise and Its Pitfalls

Like so many other innovations, digital technologies—AI included—represent a mixed bag. It can complicate healthcare interactions through the introduction of EMRs. The design of these EMRs, along with the language embedded within them as well as their perceived lack of individual authorship, may lead to biased or misguided healthcare delivery. The emergence of social media and direct-to-consumer healthcare platforms has also complicated care in that while these outlets may promote patient autonomy and work to slowly erode medicine's paternalistic traditions, they come with their own set of risks to patient health. Social media is rife with misinformation and so providers are now faced with having to address such misinformation in their patient consultations, but to do so in a way that acknowledges and validates the patient's desire to be an active participant in their own healthcare. Social media has also expanded the scope of the provider's professional boundaries, as some providers are adopting an advocacy role, using their social media platform to address health misinformation on a broader scale. At the same time, however, social media also serves as the means by which many patients are exposed to direct-to-consumer healthcare platforms through targeted ads. The proliferance of these platforms, and patients' ease in accessing them, is redefining medicine in terms of a consumer model. Providers must now be well-versed in the advantages and disadvantages of these modes of healthcare delivery relative to traditional care in order to articulate them to patients.

Yet, on the topic of financial models, digital AI technologies may prove to reconceptualize traditional care for the better. With large hospital systems in the U.S. buying up smaller, independent practices, providers are less able to exercise their individual autonomy. But AI's ability to improve productivity may mean seeing a larger volume of patients (translating to increased revenue) without sacrificing quality of care. The use of AI in clinical settings also means that providers can implement communication-based practices like narrative medicine, which have historically been regarded as impractical due to the time costs associated with them. As narrative medicine and comparable patients-centered practices have been shown to improve health outcomes (Hojat et al., 2011), AI healthcare tools may be said to do much the same. This is also demonstrated in the case of CDS, through which AI is reducing mortality rates and improving health outcomes.

When considering the positive qualities of digital technologies in healthcare alongside the negative, providers can quickly become overwhelmed when making decisions about how to integrate such technologies within their practice, or if they should at all. But they may take comfort in the fact that they are not left to their own devices when it comes to such matters. The World Health Organization (WHO) (2024) has published a report providing guidelines on the use of AI in clinical settings, as has the American Medical Association (2023). To explore these documents in depth, refer to the "Further Reading" section at the end of this chapter. However, through a robust education in the medical humanities and health communication, clinicians will be well-prepared to navigate such ethical quandaries. The following chapter, Chapter 7, extends this discussion of ethics by equipping providers with ethical principles that can be implemented in the context of digital technologies and several others.

Further Reading

1 The WHO's report, "Ethics and Governance of Artificial Intelligence for Health," may be accessed here: https://www.who.int/publications/i/item/9789240084759?
2 The American Medical Association's issued guidance on AI use for healthcare can be accessed here: https://www.ama-assn.org/system/files/ama-ai-principles.pdf

Multimedia Resources

1 To learn more about predictive AI in medicine, view this video on the JAMA Network: https://www.youtube.com/watch?v=MeyOIrXgnLY
2 To learn more about stigmatizing language in the EMR, listen to this interview with Dr. Mary Catherine Beach in collaboration with the Icahn School of Medicine at Mount Sinai: https://www.youtube.com/watch?v=9cmApXKJZ6Q

Questions for Reflection

1 Many healthcare providers establish a social media presence to perform advocacy work. Nurse John (@nurse.johnnn), for example, uses his platform to back nursing union strikes and fair labor practices. Dr. Jen Gunter (@drjengunter) uses her robust following to draw attention to women's health issues. Do you think leveraging a social media presence in this way is within the scope of the professional boundaries of the provider?
2 Outside of the ways that AI is presently being incorporated into healthcare, do you see any other possibilities for its integration? What problems exist in medicine that may be effectively addressed with a digital solution?
3 Do you ever see an occasion where AI could reasonably act in place of a human provider? Under what circumstances could this occur? What conditions would need to be met?

Glossary

- **Electronic medical record (EMR)**
- **Poor historian**
- **Diagnostic momentum**
- **Chart lore**
- **Resource stewardship**
- **Fee-for-service financial model**
- **Multi-payer system**
- **Single-payer system**
- **Underinsured**
- **Deductible**
- **Relative value units (RVUs)**

Notes

1 Resource stewardship refers to the ethical obligation to responsibly utilize healthcare resources by recommending only those tests and treatments that are evidence-based and likely to benefit the patient while avoiding unnecessary interventions that may increase costs or risks.

2 The first author of this article is featured in an interview at the end of this chapter, where he discusses the advantages and limitations of AI in medicine.

References

Adams, R., Henry, K. E., Sridharan, A., Soleimani, H., Zhan, A., Rawat, N., & Saria, S. (2022). Prospective, multi-site study of patient outcomes after implementation of the TREWS machine learning-based early warning system for sepsis. *Nature Medicine*, *28*(7), 1455–1460.

ADP Research. (2025). People at Work 2025: A global workforce view. https://assets.ctfassets.net/krliz59cjjbd/4cywXiqS7l80wNzmPXAcvT/d10903ff50927c9f-42f87a98f1b49c6a/PAW2025-Final-compressed.pdf

American Medical Association. (2023, November). *Principles for augmented intelligence development, deployment, and use*. https://www.ama-assn.org/system/files/ama-ai-principles.pdf

Bartesaghi, M., & Forbes, S. (Eds.). (2026). *Dialogues of the clinic: Encounters across medicine and beyond*. John Benjamins.

Beach, M. C., Harrigian, K., Chee, B., Ahmad, A., Links, A. R., Zirikly, A., & Saha, S. (2025). Racial bias in clinician assessment of patient credibility: Evidence from electronic health records. *PloS One*, *20*(8), e0328134.

Bryant, A. D., Fletcher, G. S., & Payne, T. H. (2014). Drug interaction alert override rates in the meaningful use era. *Applied Clinical Informatics*, *5*(3), 802–813.

Cross, S. H., & Warraich, H. J. (2021). *Rural–urban differences in mortality in the United States, 1999–2019* (NCHS Data Brief No. 417). National Center for Health Statistics, Centers for Disease Control and Prevention. https://www.cdc.gov/nchs/products/databriefs/db417.htm

Cunningham, M. (2026, February 3). *More companies are pointing to AI as they lay off employees*. CBS News. https://www.cbsnews.com/news/ai-layoffs-2026-artificial-intelligence-amazon-pinterest/

Ding, K., Forbes, S., Ma, F., Luo, G., Zhou, J., & Qi, Y. (2024). AI bias in lung cancer radiotherapy. *Exploration of Digital Health Technologies*, *2*(6), 302–312.

Forbes, S. (2015). Measuring disability: The agency of an attention deficit/hyperactivity disorder diagnostic questionnaire. *Discourse Studies*, *17*(1), 25–40.

Georgetown University Health Policy Institute. (n.d.). Rural and urban health. Georgetown University. https://hpi.georgetown.edu/rural/

Goffman, I. (1974). *Frame analysis: An essay on the organization of experience*. Harvard University Press.

Gomes, R. G., Vwalika, B., Lee, C., Willis, A., Sieniek, M., Price, J. T., & Shetty, S. (2022). A mobile-optimized artificial intelligence system for gestational age and fetal malpresentation assessment. *Communications Medicine*, *2*(1), 128.

Goody, J. (1986). *The logic of writing and the organization of society*. Cambridge University Press.

Hibbard, J. H., & Greene, J. (2013). What the evidence shows about patient activation: Better health outcomes and care experiences; fewer data on costs. *Health Affairs*, *32*(2), 207–214.

Hojat, M., Louis, D. Z., Markham, F. W., Wender, R., Rabinowitz, C., & Gonnella, J. S. (2011). Physicians' empathy and clinical outcomes for diabetic patients. *Academic Medicine*, *86*(3), 359–364.

Ilgen, J. S., & Dhaliwal, G. (2025). Educational strategies to prepare trainees for clinical uncertainty. *New England Journal of Medicine*, *393*(16), 1624–1632.

Kane, L. (2020, January 15). Medscape National Physician Burnout & Suicide Report 2020: The Generational Divide. Medscape. https://www.medscape.com/slideshow/2020-lifestyle-burnout-6012460

Kim, J., Youm, H., Kim, S., Choi, H., Kim, D., Shin, S., & Chung, J. (2024). Exploring the influence of YouTube on digital health literacy and health exercise intentions: The role of parasocial relationships. *Behavioral Sciences*, *14*(4), 282.

Latour, B. (1987). *Science in action: How to follow scientists and engineers through society*. Harvard University Press.

Leiserowitz, G., Mansfield, J., MacDonald, S., & Jost, M. (2025). Patient attitudes toward ambient voice technology: Preimplementation patient survey in an academic medical center. *JMIR Medical Informatics*, *13*(1), e77901.

McCarthy, J., Minsky, M. L., Rochester, N., & Shannon, C. E. (2006). A proposal for the Dartmouth summer research project on artificial intelligence, August 31, 1955. *AI Magazine*, *27*(4), 12.

McCrear, S. (2025, August 13). *Electronic health records suggest racial bias in assessment of patients' claims. The American Journal of Managed Care*. https://www.ajmc.com/view/electronic-health-records-suggest-racial-bias-in-assessment-of-patients-claims?

McLuhan, M. (1964). *Understanding media: The extensions of man*. McGraw-Hill.

Medscape. (2020, January 15). *National physician burnout & suicide report 2020* (Physician Lifestyle & Happiness Report). Medscape. https://www.medscape.com/slideshow/2020-lifestyle-burnout-6012460?faf=1

Ogdie, A. R., Reilly, J. B., Pang, W. G., Keddem, S., Barg, F. K., Von Feldt, J. M., & Myers, J. S. (2012). Seen through their eyes: Residents' reflections on the cognitive and contextual components of diagnostic errors in medicine. *Academic Medicine*, *87*(10), 1361–1367.

Park, J., Saha, S., Chee, B., Taylor, J., & Beach, M. C. (2021). Physician use of stigmatizing language in patient medical records. *JAMA Network Open*, *4*(7), e2117052.

Pollard, M. S., & Davis, L. M. (2022). Decline in trust in the centers for disease control and prevention during the COVID-19 pandemic. *Rand Health Quarterly*, *9*(3), 23.

Sims, R., Michaleff, Z. A., Glasziou, P., & Thomas, R. (2021). Consequences of a diagnostic label: A systematic scoping review and thematic framework. *Frontiers in Public Health*, *9*, 725877.

Skinner, A. C., & Slifkin, R. T. (2007). Rural/urban differences in barriers to and burden of care for children with special health care needs. *The Journal of Rural Health*, *23*(2), 150–157.

The Commonwealth Fund. (2024, November 21). *State of health insurance coverage in the U.S.* https://www.commonwealthfund.org/publications/surveys/2024/nov/state-health-insurance-coverage-us-2024-biennial-survey

Tun, H. M., Rahman, H. A., Naing, L., & Malik, O. A. (2025). Trust in AI-based clinical decision support systems among healthcare workers: A systematic review. *Journal of Medical Internet Research*, *10*, 69678.

Underdahl, L., Ditri, M., & Duthely, L. M. (2024). Physician burnout: Evidence-based roadmaps to prioritizing and supporting personal wellbeing. *Journal of Healthcare Leadership*, 15–27. https://doi.org/10.2147/JHL.S389245

Vanka, A., Johnston, K. T., Delbanco, T., DesRoches, C. M., Garcia, A., Salmi, L., & Blease, C. (2025). Guidelines for patient-centered documentation in the era of open notes: Qualitative study. *JMIR Medical Education*, *11*(1), e59301.

Venkat, K. K. (2015). Short and sweet: Writing better consult notes in the era of the electronic medical record. *Cleveland Clinic Journal of Medicine*, *82*(1), 13–17.
Wang, C., Tang, D., Liu, J., Zhang, S., Xu, Y., Qiao, J., & Cao, Y. (2022). Association between COVID-19 vaccination and artificial insemination outcomes for couples experiencing infertility. *JAMA Network Open*, *5*(12), e2247216.
Weick, K. E. (1995). *Sensemaking in organizations*. Sage Publications.
Willard-Grace, R., Knox, M., Huang, B., Hammer, H., Kivlahan, C., & Grumbach, K. (2019). Burnout and health care workforce turnover. *The Annals of Family Medicine*, *17*(1), 36–41.
Wong, A., Otles, E., Donnelly, J. P., Krumm, A., McCullough, J., DeTroyer-Cooley, O., & Singh, K. (2021). External validation of a widely implemented proprietary sepsis prediction model in hospitalized patients. *JAMA Internal Medicine*, *181*(8), 1065–1070.
World Health Organization. (2024). Ethics and governance of artificial intelligence for health: Guidance on large multimodal models (AI Ethics & Governance Guidance). https://www.who.int/publications/i/item/9789240084759

7 Navigating Conversations at End of Life

The Final Word

Bioethics at the End of Life

In 1998, a group of Florida physicians found themselves embroiled in what would turn into a landmark debate among medical providers, the patient's family, the media, the then-governor of Florida, the Catholic Church, and even each other. This case was that of Terri Schiavo (Figure 7.1).

On February 25, 1990, then-26-year-old Terri Schiavo collapsed in her St. Petersburg, Florida home due to cardiac arrest. Various news agencies reporting on the incident indicated that the proximate cause of her heart failure was hypokalemia brought on by an eating disorder (Weijer, 2005). Schiavo was discovered by her husband, Michael, who then called 911. Schiavo was anoxic until help arrived, and ultimately stabilized into a persistent vegetative state. Without an **advance directive** in place, her husband and parents vehemently disagreed about Terri's wishes regarding end-of-life care. Schiavo's husband argued that she would not want to be on prolonged life support, which would sustain her through artificial means; her parents, Robert and Mary Schindler, claimed the opposite. Advanced directives "are legal documents that outline an individual's preferences regarding major medical decisions" (House et al., 2025). Without such a document in place, Michael Schiavo and the Schindlers turned to the courts to adjudicate over the matter. The resulting court case became a seven-year battle, and one that garnered the attention of national media, then-Florida Governor Jeb Bush, and even the Vatican, the latter two of which adopted a Pro-Life stance with regard to the case.

In 2003, Bush helped enact "Terri's Law," which allows for state intervention in medical decision-making, and in Schiavo's specific case, authorized the reinsertion of her feeding tube despite court orders in place mandating its removal. The law was eventually overturned, however, as the Florida Supreme Court ruled it unconstitutional. Schiavo's feeding tube was once again removed and she died 13 days later on March 18, 2005 (Weijer, 2005).

While Schiavo's case became a national headline, she was by no means the first individual to become a contentious figurehead for end-of-life matters.

DOI: 10.4324/9781003654308-7

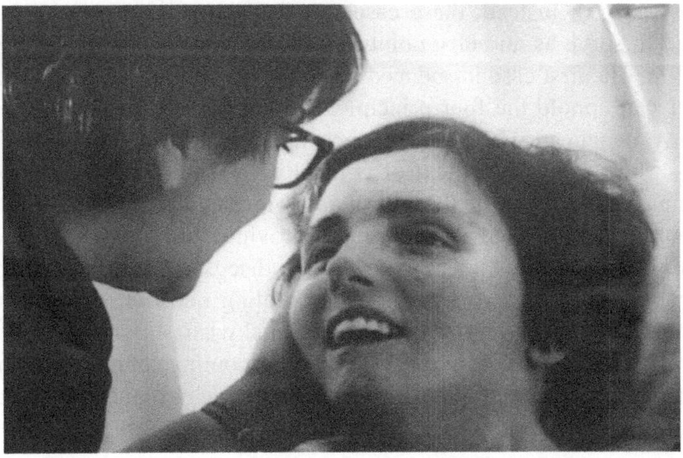

Figure 7.1 Terri Schiavo shown here in a persistent vegetative state. Photo from Getty Images.

Several decades prior, the public was forced to contemplate similar issues with the case of Margaret Ann Quinlan, who, in 1975, entered into a similar persistent vegetative state due to prolonged respiratory arrest stemming from the concurrent use of alcohol and recreational drugs. Quinlan's case represented a landmark legal case in that the New Jersey Supreme Court ruled that in the absence of an advance directive, a surrogate decision-maker could be designated for specifying the patient's end-of-life wishes (in Quinlan's case, her father) (Stonecipher, 2006). Less than ten years later, in 1983, Nancy Cruzan experienced a traumatic brain injury as the result of a car accident and then likewise entered into a persistent vegetative state (Annas, 1990). Her family petitioned the state to withdraw artificial nutrition, insisting that it undermined Cruzan's previously expressed wishes. After a long legal battle, the Supreme Court of Missouri considered new evidence in the case, including testimony from coworkers who asserted that Cruzan expressed a desire to never continue to live in such a state. Such evidence eventually prompted the Court to reverse previous rulings and ultimately resulted in the passing of the 1991 Patient Self-Determination Act, which required that hospitals, rehabilitative and nursing facilities, as well as hospice programs inform patients about their "right to make forward-looking care and treatment decisions through the use of advance directives" (Taub, 2001, p. 411).

This chapter begins by presenting a case not unlike that of Schiavo, Quinlan, and Cruzan, but it is important to specify the scope of the present discussion. The goal of the present chapter is not to deliberate on philosophical questions of life and death, consciousness or unconsciousness, and so on (e.g., "What qualifies as 'brain death'?" "What signs of life would be considered sufficient in such cases?"). Instead, these cases, as they have been presented here, are designed to serve as an entry point into the broader world of bioethics at the end of life. The first case introduced here therefore functions to consider how a provider can uphold the four principles guiding bioethical decision-making—autonomy, beneficence, non-maleficence, and justice (Beauchamp & Childress, 1979)—in the concrete context of clinical care. The next case, Case 2, more fully engages with one of these principles in particular, autonomy, but does so from the distinct perspective of the provider (as opposed to the patient only). Finally, Case 3 is intended to resume discussions initiated in the earlier chapters (Chapter 4, in particular) by prompting questions about how a provider may initiate conversations about patients' wishes around end of life. The chapter then proceeds by interrogating the shortcomings of multi-step models to communication so as to offer an alternative approach grounded in collaborative meaning-making between patient and provider.

Case 1

Patient: Mr. Bennett, aged 62, is a retired elementary school teacher with advanced amyotrophic lateral sclerosis (ALS). His primary care physician and a consulting neurologist diagnosed him nearly five years ago, and he has been experiencing aggressive functional decline ever since. He is now quadriplegic, requires oxygen support at night, and has a percutaneous endoscopic gastrostomy (PEG) tube to receive nutrition. Despite such physical deterioration, however, his cognitive functioning remains intact, and he is able to communicate in a limited fashion, using eye-tracking technology.

Scenario: Mr. Bennett has been admitted to the intensive care unit of a New England (Northeastern U.S.) hospital with aspiration pneumonia. This marks the third time he has been admitted in the course of six months. His condition has remained unresponsive to antibiotics and respiratory support, hence the reason for his being transferred to the ICU, where he can receive mechanical ventilation (Figure 7.2).

Providers: Dr. Navid Ahmadi is Mr. Bennett's attending intensivist in the Medical Intensive Care Unit. A neurologist is consulted during the admission, and so Dr. Maya Cohen is also seeing Mr. Bennett. Nurse Natalie Stevenson also cares for Mr. Bennett in the ICU.

Two years earlier, when he could still speak, Mr. Bennett completed an advance directive that specified in no uncertain terms that he would not want "artificial measures for life support in the event that recovery or a reasonable quality of life were unlikely to be achieved." His wife, Sarah, is both his power of attorney, entrusted with legal decision-making on his behalf, and his healthcare proxy.

During his most recent hospital stay, Mr. Bennett has continuously communicated through the use of his eye-tracking device that he wishes to transition

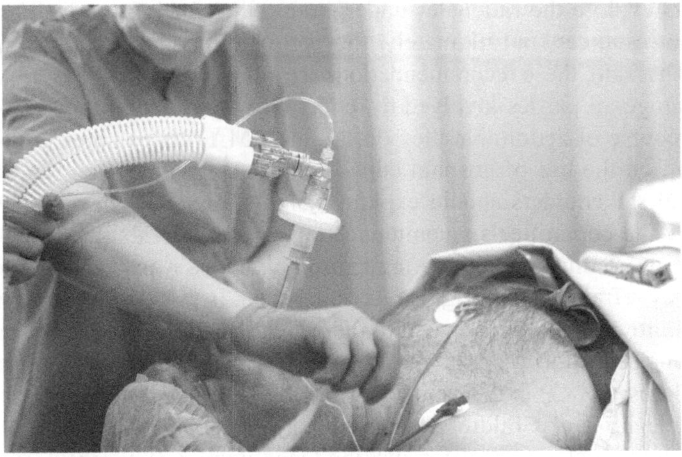

Figure 7.2 A man being intubated. Photo from Shutterstock.

to palliative care and discontinue respiratory support. He has stated, "I can't keep doing this. I just want to go in peace."

Mrs. Bennett, however, strongly opposes this plan, arguing that removing the ventilator would amount to causing her husband's death. She underscores that, as Christians, they believe the timing of Mr. Bennett's death is for God to decide, not individual patients or providers. The Bennetts' adult daughter aligns with her mother's position, whereas their adult son favors his father's perspective.

Mr. Bennett's clinical care team (detailed above) has called in the hospital's **ethics committee** to consult on the legal liabilities and ethical entailments of this conflict.

Dr. Ahmadi believes that continued ventilation is unlikely to alter Mr. Bennett's prognosis and therefore not worth pursuing. Dr. Cohen adopts a similar position, contending that Mr. Bennett's condition will only deteriorate. Mr. Bennett's ICU nurse, Nurse Natalie Stevenson, has indicated to the team that she feels moral distress about continuing a treatment plan that appears to directly contradict Mr. Bennett's stated wishes.

The Four Pillars of Ethical Decision-Making in Healthcare

Case 1 introduces two new terms worth unpacking here, the first of which is an ethics committee. Many providers are unaware that such a team exists and therefore equally unaware of the support this team of different personnel specializing in bioethics can often provide. In their definition of ethics committees, American Medical Association (2026) is careful to frame ethics committees as advisors and educators rather than decision-makers. They can help patients and providers explore the rationales underpinning their beliefs, as well as suggest available resources, but ultimately, they provide recommendations, not judgments. That said, these recommendations are influential in that they are designed to encourage all parties involved to reflect on why it is that they want to pursue the course of action that they do. As the AMA (2026) notes in its opinion statement on the use of hospital ethics committees, "Physicians and other institutional stakeholders should explain their reasoning when they choose not to follow the committee's recommendations in an individual case." So, while the hospital's ethics committee may strongly advise a particular action to be taken, they refrain from outright prescribing such. In this way, the hospital's ethics committee aims to preserve both the patient's and the provider's autonomy, which represents the first principle of the four principles outlined by Beauchamp and Childress (1979) in their model of bioethical decision-making.

Beauchamp and Childress are credited with pioneering the **principalist approach** to bioethical decision-making (see Figure 7.3), wherein, simply put, those involved in making such decisions use ethical principles to guide them. The first of these principles is "**respect for autonomy**." This means recognizing that individuals with adequate **decisional capacity**, who have expressed **informed consent** (refer to Chapter 2), are competent to make decisions about their own healthcare. It is with regard to both the issues of decisional capacity and informed consent, however, that unilaterally upholding these principles across health contexts becomes difficult.

Decisional capacity itself is determined by four fundamental abilities as demonstrated by the patient (Grisso & Appelbaum, 1998). The first ability a patient must demonstrate to be said to have decisional capacity is understanding. To be able to possess decisional capacity, the patient must be able to properly interpret the information surrounding their case, including their diagnosis, the

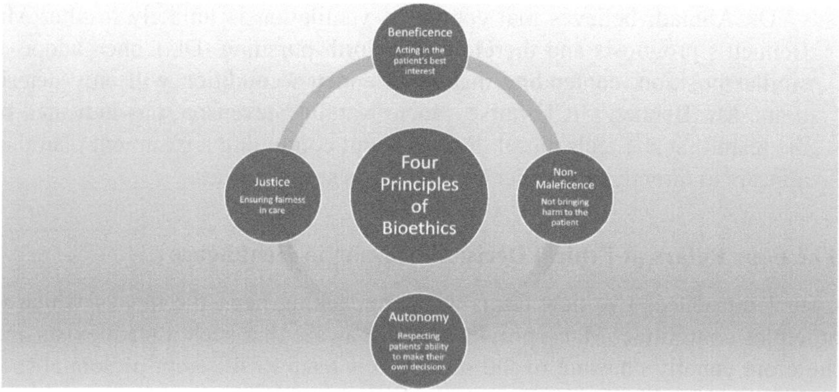

Figure 7.3 The four principles of bioethical decision-making (Beauchamp & Childress, 1979). Figure was author-generated.

proposed treatment plans, and the risks and benefits attached. The next criterion a patient must meet to possess decisional capacity is appreciation. This means that the patient is not only able to understand the information being conveyed to them, but can adequately apply it to their own situation. Next is reasoning, meaning that the patient is able to weigh risks and benefits and properly think through the entailments of what they have been told. Finally, a patient must be able to clearly communicate their decision, and that decision must remain consistent over time.

As to where decisional capacity intersects with informed consent, the former is essentially a requisite for the latter. One cannot provide informed consent—that is, voluntary authorization to participate in a medical intervention—without meeting the conditions of decisional capacity. In cases like Terri Schiavo's, upholding the principle of autonomy became difficult precisely because she did not have the decisional capacity to provide informed consent. Mr. Bennett's case is quite different, however. In examining the four core components of decisional capacity, it becomes clear that Mr. Bennett meets all of the specified criteria. Mr. Bennett understands both his diagnosis and poor prognosis; he appreciates that continued ventilation is unlikely to change this prognosis; he has reasoned through the value he assigns to quality of life versus longevity; and finally, he communicates a consistent choice using his eye-tracking software. Mr. Bennett's continued refusal of mechanical ventilation thus signals informed consent, which, importantly, may be expressed through nonverbal means, as in this case.

When taken together, Mr. Bennett's evidence of decisional capacity and his ability to provide informed consent indicate that providers must strive to uphold his autonomy in medical decision-making. From a health communication perspective, however, the question then becomes one of how best to do that.

To start, the involved providers should grant equal weight to various modes of communication. In legal contexts, greater authority is conferred to nonverbal forms of communication expressed in writing. Yet, in healthcare contexts, less formal means should also be carefully considered. For example, Mr. Bennett's communication via assistive technologies should not be interpreted as less compelling than that which may be conveyed in an advance directive or what he might otherwise state orally if he could. This recommendation becomes especially important if a patient expresses wishes through one mode of communication (for example, orally, in person) that appears to contradict an earlier declaration (for example, that which is stated in an advance directive). Such contradictions could compromise decisional capacity, as the fourth criterion specifies that the indicated decision must remain stable.

With regard to Mr. Bennett's mode of communication, specifically, providers should also open up the conversational floor for the patient to communicate their wishes fully and at length. Patients like Mr. Bennett, who have physical impairments, may need more time to express themselves. Providers may help "hold the floor" for patients in similar positions by gently discouraging other parties from interjecting. This might look as simple as stating something like, "This sounds like a great point, one I'd like to revisit a bit more after Mr. Bennett finishes what he was saying."

Another way that providers can aim to uphold Mr. Bennett's autonomy through their communication practices is by speaking to him before other family members. This simple act acknowledges that Mr. Bennett is still the primary decision-maker when it comes to his own health matters, and therefore will be consulted first. Relatedly, providers may also choose to reinforce this position by verbally underscoring the primacy of Mr. Bennett's contributions to the conversation with statements like, "As Mr. Bennett has repeatedly expressed" or "Mr. Bennett has indicated on several occasions." Such declarations should also be documented in his medical record so that they can be similarly referenced by other members of the care team for consistent communication across various channels.

It is worth pointing out that in their discussions of autonomy for ethical decision-making, Beauchamp and Childress only apply it to the concept to the patient. Little to nothing is said of the provider's autonomy. The fact that Nurse Stevenson feels moral distress over the debate surrounding Mr. Bennett's continued care points to providers' autonomy in medical decision-making. **Moral distress** often results from the tension between knowing the ethical course of action and feeling unable to pursue it due to institutional or pragmatic constraints. In Nurse Stevenson's case, she experiences moral distress presumably because she feels that continuing ventilation despite Mr. Bennett's indication that he wishes to do otherwise would be a violation of his autonomy. She may feel constrained to act, however, as she is not the attending supervising his care, nor is she the only member of his care team.

Providers often experience moral distress when they believe their actions are undermining the next two principles of Beauchamp and Childress's (1979) four-part model, which are often treated as two sides of the same coin. These principles are **beneficence** and **non-maleficence**. "Beneficence" refers to the ethical obligation to operate for the benefit of others. In a similar vein, "non-maleficence" would be more in line with the "do no harm" injunction so prevalent in medicine. How these two principles apply to Mr. Bennett's case appears fairly straightforward. Continued mechanical ventilation in light of the patient's expressed desire for otherwise violates both principles. This course of action will provide little to no benefit to him (compromising beneficence), as both Drs. Ahmadi and Cohen indicate in their assessment of the situation. In fact, it is more likely to cause harm to him (undermining non-maleficence), as he may incur unnecessary emotional distress and physical discomfort due to the prolonged ventilation. Indeed, this discomfort may eventually extend into more overt risks to his health, including ventilator-associated pneumonia (VAP), tracheal damage and stenosis, and diaphragm atrophy, just to name a few.

The final principle to consider in Mr. Bennett's case is **justice**. The principle of justice moves from solely considering the individual themselves to reflect on broader social forces and how said forces affect matters of health equity. Questioning justice in healthcare decision-making entails questioning equitable access to healthcare, the fair distribution of healthcare resources, and the delivery of impartial care, regardless of the patient's race, gender, socioeconomic or health status, and so on. In Mr. Bennett's case, justice comes into play when one considers that healthcare resources are finite. Supplying a ventilator to Mr. Bennett, despite his expressed wishes against this, may mean this resource is not available to another patient who has indicated in explicit terms that they elect to receive such an intervention. Therefore, in light of considerations for justice, one can see how the other three principles intersect in an independent fashion; because Mr. Bennett's autonomy is not being upheld, justice is called into question, as is the potential harm and benefit brought to him and other patients. For a detailed depiction of these principles in relation to one another, refer to Figure 7.3.

Case 2

Patient: Ms. Alexa Rossi, 41, is a high school math teacher living in British Columbia. She was first diagnosed with treatment-resistant major depressive disorder (MDD) at the age of 22. For nearly two decades, she has sought various forms of treatment in the forms of pharmacological solutions, electroconvulsive therapy (ECT), and inpatient psychiatric hospitalizations and rehabilitation facilities. Despite these various interventions, however, Ms. Rossi has not witnessed a significant reduction in her symptoms.

While Ms. Rossi claims that her condition exerts several negative impacts on her life, she is fully independent in her daily life. She also possesses full cognitive abilities.

Ms. Rossi is accompanied on her visit to her psychiatrist's office today by her partner of 12 years, Jordan Garcia. Mr. Garcia and Ms. Rossi are not legally married, but cohabitate, and have no children (Figure 7.4).

Scenario: Ms. Rossi has come to see the psychiatrist who has been following her for the past eight years to inquire about Canada's Medical Assistance in Dying (MAiD) program, which has recently (as of 2021) expanded eligibility criteria for participation in this program to include Axis 1 psychiatric disorders as sufficiently qualifying patients for the program under certain conditions.

After discussing what MAiD entails with her psychiatrist, Ms. Rossi states, "I'm not confused. I've thought about this for a long time now. We don't make dogs and cats suffer when they are chronically ill. Why can't I be afforded the same courtesy? I have lived with this illness most of my adult life; I don't want to do so any longer."

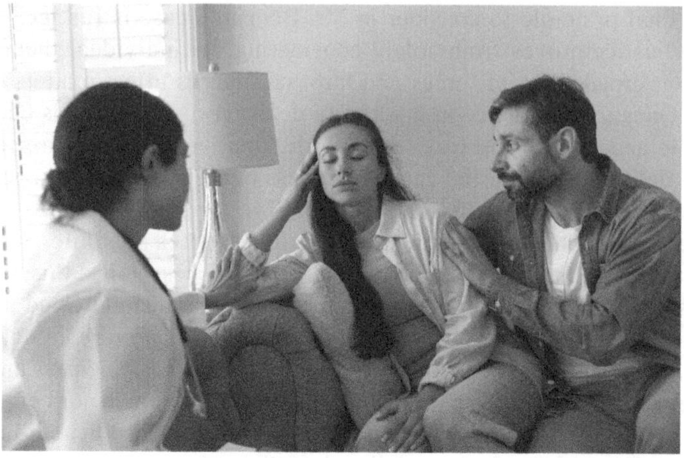

Figure 7.4 A young woman in distress, accompanied by her partner. Photo from Shutterstock.

Ms. Rossi has undergone extensive psychiatric evaluations for decisional capacity. All of these assessments indicate that she offers a consistent rationale and is fully aware of the implications of her decision. Psychiatric notes also indicate that she is not acutely suicidal.

Mr. Garcia believes this decision to be consistent with Ms. Rossi's core beliefs regarding autonomy, dignity, and the right to be free of suffering. Ms. Garcia corroborates Ms. Rossi's story that this decision is not sudden, and one that they have discussed on many occasions throughout the years of their relationship.

Ms. Rossi's younger brother and parents, all of whom live in Ontario, are vehemently opposed to this decision. They argue that depression is a treatable condition and that authorizing her request creates a "slippery slope" for other non-terminal illnesses to be used as a grounds for MAiD. Communication between Ms. Rossi, Mr. Garcia, and Ms. Rossi's family have become strained, with her family threatening to pursue legal recourse.

Providers: Dr. Francois Tremblay is Ms. Rossi's psychiatrist, who has followed Ms. Rossi for the past eight years. Dr. Tremblay admits that Ms. Rossi's case does technically meet the criteria for MAiD, but is morally conflicted over participating in MAiD. Dr. Tremblay believes, like Ms. Rossi's family, that there is always the possibility of treatment success with psychiatric illness. Dr. Tremblay has therefore decided that he will invoke conscientious objection and will refuse to serve as a MAiD assessor or provider, though he will continue to provide psychiatric care should Ms. Rossi wish.

A second psychiatrist within Dr. Tremblay's practice, Dr. Samantha Fournier, adopts a different stance, arguing that Dr. Tremblay's refusal constitutes medical paternalism and undermines patient autonomy.

To better understand the details of this case, we must first examine how this program came to be within Canada. The Medical Aid in Dying (MAiD) problem was legalized in Canada in 2016 with the Supreme Court ruling issued in the Carter v. Canada 2015 case. In this case, the court ruled that denying assisted death to those experiencing "grievous and unremediable" terminal illness violated the Canadian Charter of Rights and Freedoms. In 2021, the law was amended to remove the requirement that one's death must be imminent, thus opening the door for consideration of psychiatric disorders as grounds for MAiD. As of 2024, the law was amended yet again to temporarily exclude individuals whose sole condition for participation was psychiatric in nature, with their eligibility not expected to resume until 2027 (Government of Canada, n.d.).

The MAiD program has been extensively critiqued, particularly from the bioethical principle of justice. Prominent critics of the program, like Coelho et al. (2023) argue that the program may act in a predatory fashion for people with disabilities, those with fewer socioeconomic resources, and patients without access to medical or social support. Others like Middleton (2019), who wrote in a letter published in the *Canadian Medical Association Journal*, argue that MAiD becomes especially problematic when introduced in the same context as organ donation. She writes, "I have concerns that organ donation after MAiD has the potential to influence substantially the decision of individual patients to proceed with MAiD and also to increase the number of requests for MAiD" (p. 1062).

The Politics of a "Good" Death

Given the mixed reception MAiD has received, it is unsurprising that Dr. Tremblay feels similarly torn. The moral distress Dr. Tremblay is experiencing over Ms. Rossi's request has prompted him to refuse to participate, and to claim **conscientious objection**. Conscientious objection was traditionally applied to wartime contexts, where pacifists and members of certain religions like Quakers, Mennonites, and fundamentalist Christians refused to bear arms, claiming that doing so violated their moral, ethical, and/or religious beliefs. More recently, the use of this term has been applied to healthcare contexts, often in discussions of provider autonomy. Acknowledging a growing body of research that links provider moral distress to provider burnout and overall employment attrition in certain fields (see Buchbinder et al., 2024a, 2024b), scholars working in the medical humanities have paid special attention to how conscientious objection applies to health contexts. These scholars have posed questions like, "Under what circumstances can a provider reasonably and ethically invoke conscientious objection?" "How does the provider's right to exercise their autonomy (i.e., by refusing care) come up against a patient's right to exercise their autonomy (i.e., control of their own healthcare decision-making)?" And, "Are there situations where a provider should be prevented from invoking conscientious objection?"

Within the U.S., questions such as these have come to the fore of discussions of healthcare ethics, as shifting laws around abortion care vary state by state and moment to moment. In the U.S., where many states have total bans on abortion, including Alabama, Kentucky, Louisiana, Mississippi, Tennessee, and Texas), invoking conscientious objection may introduce an ethical dilemma. Notably, these states are located in the American South, where abortion laws are much more restrictive than throughout the country. As a result of the increasing restrictions placed on abortions in this region of the country, it becomes much more problematic when a provider refuses to provide such services, as the nearest willing provider may be a great distance away. For patients with few financial and material resources, it may not be feasible to travel such distances to obtain an abortion. It is here that the principles outlined by Beauchamp and Childress (1979) may be jeopardized. Should the provider refuse to provide care, especially in an emergent situation where a timely abortion could be life-saving, this could violate the principle of non-maleficence, or doing what will bring the least harm to patients. Additionally, one might consider how refusals in areas with few available abortion providers undermine the principle of justice because patients in specific geographic locales and those with fewer financial resources to leave do not receive the same healthcare as their counterparts. This begs the question, "What should the provider do to remain true to their own ethical and moral commitments, while continuing to promote the beneficence of the patient?"

The answer to this question typically lies in referring to another qualified provider. This has become the gold standard of care in such instances, as referring the patient to another provider ensures that they receive high-quality care, as theoretically, a provider who is morally opposed to performing some procedures may not perform them as well as someone who is not, and so that the patient does not fall victim to **systemic abandonment** (Biehl, 2005). Systemic abandonment in healthcare occurs when institutional policies and practices repeatedly prevent certain groups of patients from receiving reliable, affordable, and accessible healthcare. In the case of Dr. Tremblay, then, avoiding systemic abandonment while still exercising conscientious objection might look like referring Ms. Rossi to his colleague who holds a different view, Dr. Fournier. This way, Ms. Rossi is able to nonetheless engage in autonomous decision-making and Dr. Tremblay is able to refrain from undertaking actions that compromise his moral standards. This practice remains ethical in Ms. Rossi's case, where a nearby provider who can offer the services being denied is easily accessible.

In many ways, Ms. Rossi's case echoes aspects of the Schiavo case. While Terri Schiavo did not have the decisional capacity that Ms. Rossi does, the division among family members remains a salient issue in both instances. In both cases, the spouse or long-time partner is the one supporting the patient's wishes, whereas their blood-related kin advocate for a different course of action. The division here can be seen as falling upon the lines of **family of origin** versus **family of choice**. "Family of origin" typically refers to the family one was born into—their blood relatives. "Family of choice," as the name suggests, defines family as something other than "bio-legal bonds" (Jackson Levin et al., 2020), as the friends, spouses, partners, and so on that one *chooses* for themselves. In Ms. Rossi's case, as well as in Terri Schiavo's case, the patient's family of choice is composed of their partner and spouse, respectively, and their family of origin encompasses their parents and siblings.

Historically, medicine has failed to grant equal weight to both types of families. This was particularly evident during the HIV/AIDS epidemic of the 1980s and 1990s, where, at least in the U.S., lifelong partners and friends were systematically excluded from visitation, caregiving, or end-of-life decision-making (Figure 7.5). Instead, as Weston (1997) points out, gay patients during this time relied on friends and partners for support, but these relationships were delegitimized by medicine, which afforded primary healthcare decision-making rights to the patient's biological family members. Even against the backdrop of modern medicine, families of choice are often seen as secondary, lesser, or supplementary, but rarely as an interchangeable substitute for families of origin. This invites a perplexing question, one which asks, "In the absence of a formally designated power of attorney or healthcare proxy, what should providers do when family members cannot reach a consensus over patients' care?" In Ms. Rossi's case, how should Dr. Tremblay and any other provider involved in her care navigate the complex communication dynamics characterized by her family of choice (i.e., Mr. Garcia) advocating one thing and her family of origin (i.e., her parents and younger brother) another?

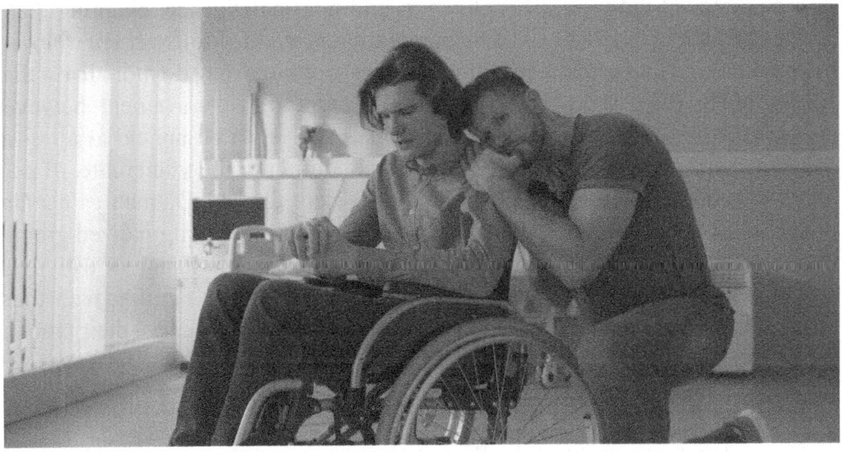

Figure 7.5 A same-sex couple consoling one another in a medical setting. Photo from Shutterstock.

The first practice providers can make a hallmark of their communication with the patient and their families is to resist organizing types of family, or even individual family members, hierarchically. This necessitates checking any implicit assumptions or latent biases that suggest that biological relations trump other types of bonds. Such a practice would moreover extend to not only to type of relation, but degree as well, meaning that input derived from a second cousin, aunt, or niece would not be regarded as carrying lesser weight than that which was offered by a mother, father, sibling, and so on.

Another recommendation for providers to effectively navigate family communication dynamics, especially at end of life, is to use consistent language across various contexts. As Chapter 3 demonstrated, it is very important not to underestimate the highly consequential nature of language. Therefore, providers would be well-advised to consider the connotations and perceptual impacts of different terminology surrounding end-of-life care. One particularly loaded term worth reflecting on is "physician-assisted suicide," especially when compared to approximate alternatives like "medical aid in dying." The former of these terms invokes the highly controversial term "suicide," which potentially characterizes the patient as suicidal, and thus immersed in an acute mental health crisis, which will presumably pass with time and/or active intervention (Hannig, 2022). The term "physician-assisted suicide" furthermore places the onus on the physician, positioning them as an agent or instrument of death. The latter term, however, places the focus on the means by which death is facilitated (i.e., "medicine" broadly conceived), not the individual agent bringing it about.

Other terms worthy of further consideration include the "Right to Die," and its conceptual counterpart, the "Right to Life." Both terms represent opposing political and ideological movements. The Right to Die movement emphasizes the principles of autonomy, beneficence, and non-maleficence, claiming that a patient has the "right" (i.e., is fundamentally entitled to) to exert control over their death, and that prolonged life-sustaining measures may do more harm than good (ten Have & Patrão Neves, 2021). The Right to Life movement, however, appeals to the sacredness of life—sacredness that must be upheld at all costs (Snyder, 2001). It also positions itself as a champion of the vulnerable, of people who might be susceptible to coercion to elect for MAiD, such as persons with disabilities, the impoverished, and members of other marginalized groups. Regardless of a provider's own personal and professional alignment with these movements and the terminology embedded therein, being familiar with these terms and all that they conjure up in the minds of others will serve their practice well. The same can also be said employing consistent terminology across settings and conversations so as to prevent confusion on behalf of the patient and their family.

One notable proponent of the Right to Die movement was Brittany Maynard. Diagnosed with the terminal diagnosis of glioblastoma at the age of 29, Maynard relocated from California to Oregon, where she could pursue a medically assisted death under Oregon's 1997 Death with Dignity Act. Maynard became a figurehead for the Right to Die movement, as she chose to greet death on her own terms. More than that, however, Maynard's case raised several questions about what constitutes a "good" death in Western societies. Part of the outrage over Maynard's decision stemmed from the fact that Maynard was a young woman only embarking on life as a newlywed; she was seen as "giving up" in her fight against the disease by not pursuing further treatment; and she was electing to die in her own home as opposed to a hospital, where she could presumably continue to receive life-sustaining care.

Ms. Rossi's case exhibits many of the same violations of Western understandings of a good death that Maynard's does: she is young; she is not pursuing further treatment, though available; and she is not leaving determinations of death up to fate or a higher power, but taking matters into her own hands. One key differentiating factor in Ms. Rossi's case is that her diagnosis is not terminal, which may provide further support for the claim that she is not succumbing to death but giving up on life. One final recommendation from a health communication perspective for the providers involved in Ms. Rossi's care would be to genuinely reflect on their own assumptions of what constitutes a "good death," and how such assumptions are culturally informed.

Referring once more to Chapter 2's discussion of the cultural components of health communication, it is important that providers acknowledge that definitions of a "good" death are not universal. While Drs. Tremblay and Fournier are practicing within a Western context, if their patient had hailed from another cultural setting, they may find themselves operating on discrepant beliefs as to what a "good" death looks like. A primary discrepancy between Western and non-Western understandings of a "good" death pertains to where death occurs. In the U.S., Canada, the U.K., and much of Europe, dying in a hospital or hospice or assisted living facility has become the norm. For those opting for such settings for death, there may be appeal in the ability of institutional facilities to manage symptoms at end of life, thus making the transition from life to death less traumatic overall.

In many other cultures throughout the world, however, this is atypical, as patients prefer to die at home in the presence of their family members. This is the view that was expressed by healthcare providers serving Indigenous communities throughout the Northern Territory of Australia. In their study of the palliative care services provided to these individuals, McGrath et al. (2006) found that a lack of respite or palliative care services in rural areas forced Indigenous Australians to relocate away from their families for end-of-life care, thus violating age-old traditions of dying on ancestral land and in the presence of their family members. Similar sentiments were expressed by patients in East Asian countries, with 13–22% of respondents throughout Japan, Taiwan, and

Korea indicating that they would prefer to die at home. Yang et al. (2025), however, indicate that there is a lack of congruence between this stated preference and what actually happens, as 80% of those surveyed died in palliative care units within hospitals. These findings underscore both the diversity in end-of-life preferences for healthcare delivery, as well as their culturally specific nature. They demonstrate that patients' desires are deeply influenced by geographic locale, institutional and legal constraints, family dynamics, and cultural norms.

When taken together, these studies not only highlight the culturally specific nature of end-of-life preferences and call back to Chapter 2 in this way, but they also encourage providers to reflect on the implicit motivation behind the prevalence of dying in institutional settings, as has become the norm throughout the West and the Global North. Certainly, some could agree that symptom control becomes more manageable in institutional settings, thus mitigating the likelihood of a "bad" death, as defined by prolonged suffering. However, as Ariès (1974) has pointed out, such societies have become accustomed to "hiding death away"—to removing it from the family home and confining it to hospital corridors and palliative care wings. The reasons for this, according to Ariès, are multiple. The rise in medicalization is one contributing factor; with the abundance of technologies available for prolonging life (e.g., ventilation and intravenous nutrition), in the event that a death occurs, it has come to be interpreted as a failure of medicine rather than a natural happening. More than that, though, Ariès argues that this practice of placing death out of sight reflects a refusal to confront our own mortality.

In his book, *Being Mortal: Medicine and What Matters in the End*, Gawande (2014) argues that this fear surfaces in conversations (or the lack thereof) between patients and providers at the end of life. Gawande asserts that providers often avoid explicit conversations around patients' prognoses, dying, and their goals for end-of-life care. He continues that the reason why providers avoid such conversations is due, in large part, to the "fallacy of giving up" (Hamblin, 2015). This fallacy supposes that to have such conversations—to acknowledge that medical intervention may not be effective or preferable—would mean that the provider is abandoning their patient. This is why, Gawande argues, when these conversations do eventually happen, they take place at a very late stage in patient care, after all curative options have been exhausted. Figure 7.6 depicts the relationship among grand social narratives such as "the fallacy of giving up" and those embedded in notions of what constitutes a "good death," and moreover details how these narratives intersect with legal stances and policy positions.

So, taking this to be true—that providers are uncomfortable having end-of-life conversations for fear of being perceived as abandoning their patient—what measures may be taken to make these conversations more commonplace? This question is the impetus behind Case 3, which illustrates a provider attempting to initiate and sustain such a conversation.

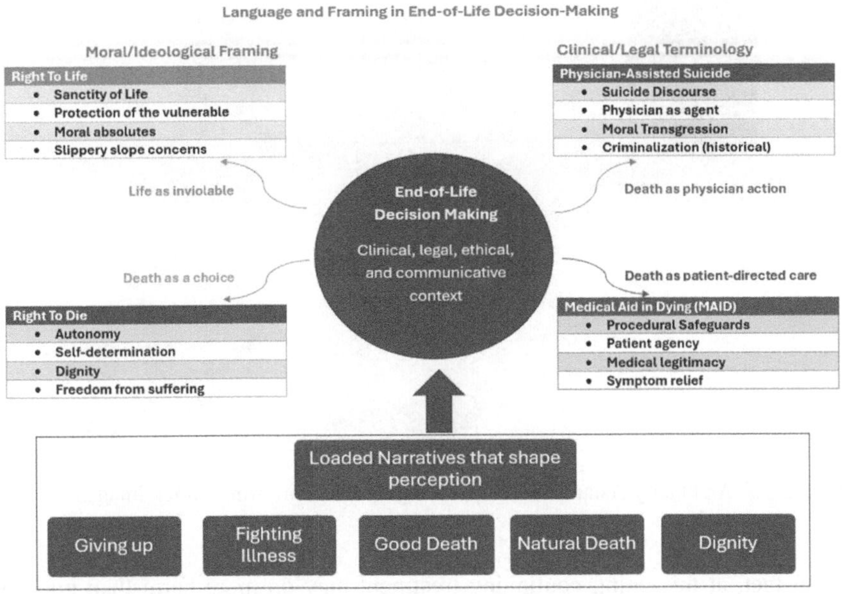

Figure 7.6 Language and moral framing in end-of-life decision-making. Image was author-generated.

Case 3

Patient: Mr. Yuri Tanaka is a 69-year-old man with stage 4 gastric cancer. He has demonstrated decisional capacity, speaks fluent English, and has been undergoing treatment for the past 12 months in the form of second-line chemotherapy. Imaging, however, suggests that his body is no longer responding to treatment as evidenced by disease progression. Mr. Tanaka lives with his wife of 40 years in nearby Hamburg, Germany, and is close with his two adult children.

Provider: Dr. Luis Wanner is a medical oncologist practicing at the University of Hamburg-Eppendorf, a large academic medical center and teaching hospital. Dr. Wanner has been an attending at the hospital for eight years now, and is known for his straightforward communication style.

Scenario: During this visit, Dr. Wanner plans to review the results of Mr. Tanaka's most recent CT scan (Figure 7.7). As Dr. Wanner enters the consult room, he pulls up a rolling stool to sit face-to-face and eye level with Mr. Tanaka, saying, "I want to review your scan results with you today. Can you tell me what you understand about your disease and how your body is responding to treatment?"

Mr. Tanaka replies, "I know that the last treatment might have not cured me, but I was hopeful it could buy me some time."

Dr. Wanner says, "I see." He continues by saying, "I want to be honest. The cancer is progressing and further regimens are unlikely to halt its advancement.

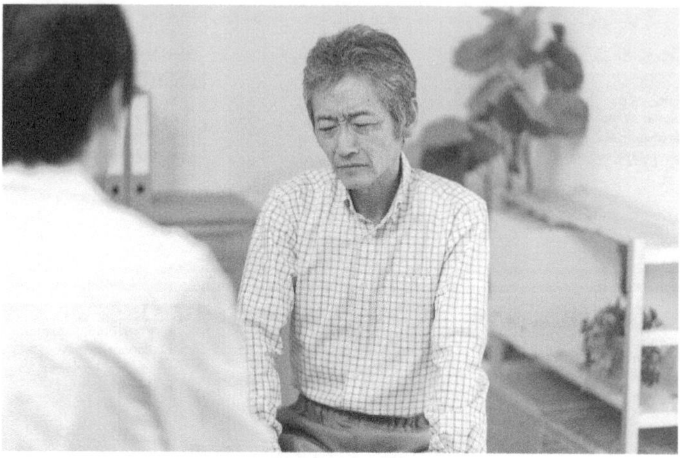

Figure 7.7 An elderly Asian patient appearing upset. Photo from iStock images.

In fact, at this point, continuing treatment may do more harm than good in terms of adverse effects. I will be sending a referral for a member of our palliative care team to discuss next steps with you."

Mr. Tanaka questions, "Is there nothing else we can do? A clinical trial, perhaps?"

After a brief moment of silence, Dr. Wanner says, "There's a lot we can do to make you comfortable. Many patients seek out our hospice services to help with this difficult transition." Noticing tears welling in his eyes, Dr. Wanner hands Mr. Tanaka a tissue and asks, "Do you have any other questions?"

Mr. Tanaka asks hesitantly, "How long do you think I have? I just don't know how my family will handle this."

Dr. Wanner offers a cautious estimate of six months, but emphasizes that no one can predict this timeline with certainty. He asks if there is anyone he can call to come be with Mr. Tanaka. He inputs the request for a hospice referral and books a follow-up appointment for Mr. Tanaka, before thanking him and exiting the room.

Breaking Bad News

Dr. Wanner's approach to this interaction with Mr. Tanaka loosely adheres to the **SPIKES model** referenced in Chapter 4. To review, the SPIKES Model for Breaking Bad News, as established by Baile et al. (2000), is a process-driven approach to healthcare communication; the provider is expected to progressively move through the various stages of breaking bad news as represented by this acronym. Referring to the "S" in the SPIKES model, setting, Dr. Wanner does well to create an ideal setting for the delivery of this information. He closes the door behind him to ensure privacy and sits face-to-face at eye level to both indicate to Mr. Tanaka that he has his full attention, and to minimize the symbolic construction of a power differential that is implied by standing over the patient. As for the "P" in the SPIKES model, perception, Dr. Wanner does inquire into Mr. Tanaka's understanding of his condition and prognosis (e.g., "Can you tell me what you understand about your disease and how your body is responding to treatment?"). However, he does not probe Mr. Tanaka's response of "I know that the last treatment might have not cured me, but I was hopeful it could buy me some time." What does "some time" mean for Mr. Tanaka? And how might culturally specific notions of time, as well as individual understandings of what constitutes "some time," influence Mr. Tanaka's use of this phrase? Is "some time" six years, six months, or six weeks? The trouble here is that failing to inquire further about how Mr. Tanaka has operationalized this expression means that Dr. Wanner has assumed mutual understanding where it may be altogether absent. Furthermore, while he has gauged the patient's perception of his condition, he has done so in a rather narrow way.

This failure represents one of the primary critiques of the SPIKES model and other process-driven approaches just like it. Operating on the assumption that if one moves through these stages in order, they will achieve the predictable, desired result of shared understanding, this model reinforces the transmission model of communication discussed in Chapter 4. The goal, however, for any provider skilled in health communication, would be to engender shared meaning through a back-and-forth exchange. In this context, that might look like Dr. Wanner asking, "What does 'some time' look like for you?" Pausing to ask this simple question would provide the opportunity to clarify any misconceptions and for the patient to express their hopes and fears surrounding end-of-life care in more explicit terms.

As for the "I" in the SPIKES model, the invitation, while Dr. Wanner announces his intention to discuss Mr. Tanaka's CT results, the invitation from the patient to proceed is minimal at best. In fact, Dr. Wanner's statement, "I want to review your scan results with you today," is much more in line with a declaration than an invitation. Unfortunately, structuring the statement in this way may work to exacerbate the power asymmetries already inherent in the provider-patient relationship, as it indicates what the provider alone would like to have happen. Furthermore, Mr. Tanaka's response, his silence, does not supply sufficient consent to proceed. In accordance with the transmission model of communication, Mr. Tanaka is treated as a passive recipient of communication, not an active participant within the encounter. A simple rephrasing in the form of "Would it be okay for me to discuss these results with you?" reframes this characterization of the patient as the recipient and provides a deliberate space for the patient to verbally confirm or deny their receipt of the invitation.

The next step of the SPIKES model, knowledge, is met, but in a perfunctory way. Dr. Wanner is careful not to employ jargon that may obscure the patient's understanding, but he nonetheless takes for granted Mr. Tanaka's knowledge of what abstract terms like "harm," "good," and "adverse effects" mean in this context. To better fulfill this criteria, and move toward the shared meaning-making endorsed by a constitutive model of communication (see Chapter 1), Dr. Wanner could explicitly invite Mr. Tanaka's take on these terms through the use of a question like, "What would a 'good' outcome look like given what I've told you?" Or, "Do you know what I mean by 'adverse effects'?" "Would it be more helpful if I detailed some of these effects for you?" Posing such questions acknowledges the two-way nature of communication, seeing meaning as something that is created together rather than received.

For these same reasons, Dr. Wanner may also wish to explore Mr. Tanaka's question, "Is there nothing else we can do? A clinical trial, perhaps?" Rather than interpret this question as purely information-seeking and respond with a simple yes/no answer, Dr. Wanner may gently inquire into the fallacy of giving up here. He may ask why Mr. Tanaka wants to pursue a clinical trial, even if it is unlikely to change his prognosis. He may explore how the fallacy enters into Mr. Tanaka's reasoning, asking if Mr. Tanaka views declining treatment as abandonment, a perceived moral deficit such as a lack of resiliency, or not placing enough value on his life as it is. Asking questions like these would better enable Dr. Wanner to provide end-of-life care that fundamentally aligns with the patient's values.

Empathy, the "E" in the SPIKES acronym, comes across as equally formulaic. Dr. Wanner does signal empathy by offering Mr. Tanaka a tissue, thus acknowledging his emotional distress, and offers to call someone, presumably his family, to be with him. But this comes across as rote. Mr. Tanaka expresses concern for what this news will do to his family, yet Dr. Wanner glosses over this, only choosing to respond to the question embedded in Mr. Tanaka's contribution. To better demonstrate empathy, Dr. Wanner could both name the emotions Mr. Tanaka is feeling and restate what it is he thinks he is hearing as a way to convey active engagement. Saying something like, "I hear how worried you are and how deeply you care for your family," names emotions Mr. Tanaka is experiencing (here, worry and care), and in doing so, validates them. This restatement further signals that Dr. Wanner is actively listening to Mr. Tanaka in a way that only responding to half his statement fails to do.

Finally, as it relates to this healthcare communication model, the "S" in SPIKES stands for both "summarize" and "strategy." Dr. Wanner does a fair job of strategizing, by detailing next steps in the form of a hospice referral and follow-up visit, but he fails to summarize the interaction. Summary becomes especially important when delivering bad news such as this because patients often experience difficulty processing information when they are emotionally overwhelmed. Receiving grave news is often extremely disorienting for patients. As Frank (1995) points out in *The Wounded Storyteller*, illness represents a break in the narrative coherence of our life's story. After receiving such information, patients and providers are tasked with allowing that story to continue, but on different terms. Summarizing the story thus far therefore represents a key juncture in allowing it to continue—in allowing the patient to resituate themselves in a disrupted narrative and make sense of what comes next.

As this case demonstrates, the SPIKES model is not wholly bad. In going through the model, Dr. Wanner has attempted to ensure that certain necessary elements of effective communication are present; he gauges the patient's existing knowledge on the subject, and he normalizes Mr. Tanaka's response by referencing other patients in a similar situation. That said, the protocol-driven nature of the SPIKES model leaves much to be desired, which is why subsequent variations have since been developed. One such variant is the COMFORT model—communication, orientation and opportunity, mindful presence, family, oversight, reiterative messages, and team (Wittenberg et al., 2018). Similar to the SPIKES model, the COMFORT model was designed for use in oncological settings, but was specifically tailored to nursing. The COMFORT model builds upon SPIKES by introducing family into the communicative equation—something that Dr. Wanner overlooks here. It furthermore broadens its view of communication beyond the dyad (i.e., the patient and provider) to include all members of the care team, as evidenced by the "T" in the model. While both the SPIKES model and the COMFORT model are helpful in that they offer some guidance for navigating an interaction that may otherwise be overwhelming for clinicians and patients alike, much gets lost on account of their goal-driven nature. Opportunities for collaboratively negotiating meaning remain unpursued, as do those for creating a plan of care that reflects the patient's values and understanding of a "good" death.

Making Meaning at End of Life

Collectively, the cases presented in this chapter speak to how end-of-life decision-making is rarely the product of a single patient's choice. These decisions are weighed against the backdrop of the societal values ascribed to life and death, and medicine's right to adjudicate over and intervene in these matters. The historical cases of Quinlan, Cruzan, and Schiavo demonstrate how these values are never settled, perpetually in flux, and constantly up for negotiation, as patients, providers, and their families are drawn into legal, ethical, and moral dilemmas. Case 1 grounds this dilemma squarely in the concrete context of the clinic by employing Mr. Bennett's experiences to illustrate decisional capacity as well as the four principles of bioethical decision-making.

Case 2 elaborates on the discussion of autonomy introduced by Case 1, this time, exploring the concept from the provider's perspective. This discussion offers a point of entry into how culturally informed assumptions guide both patients' and providers' approaches to death. In a callback to Chapter 3, it interrogates the language surrounding death, questioning how this affects perceptions of it. It moreover reflects on the narratives embedded in death, such as the fallacy of giving up, and how these influence where death occurs, under what circumstances, and as initiated by whom.

Finally, Case 3 concludes the discussion of communication at the end of life by adopting a "how-to" framework, but it does so in a way that is skeptical of an exclusively process-driven approach. It provides insight into how model-based approaches to end-of-life communication implicitly uphold a transmission-based view of communication, and in doing so, paint the patient as a passive recipient of information. Yet, by identifying "missed opportunities," it shows providers how they can move toward a more collaborative paradigm. Ultimately, the task that lays before the provider at the patient's end of life amounts to much more than going through a series of steps or using the correct language. It is a back-and-forth negotiation, a mutual undertaking, and a conversation that gives meaning to a patient's life as well as their death.

Glossary

- **Advance directive**
- **Ethics committee**
- **Principalist approach**
- **Respect for autonomy**
- **Decisional capacity**
- **Informed consent**
- **Moral distress**
- **Beneficence**
- **Non-maleficence**
- **Justice**
- **Conscientious objection**
- **Systemic abandonment**
- **Family of origin**
- **Family of choice**
- **SPIKES model**

Further Reading

1 For a slightly less academic exploration of a physician reflecting on their own mortality, read the best-selling novel/memoir *When Breath Becomes Air*: https://www.amazon.com/When-Breath-Becomes-Paul-Kalanithi/dp/081298840X

Exercises

1 As this chapter has established, many high-profile cases surrounding end-of-life decision-making escalated to such a degree of visibility due to the absence of an advance directive. Often, people think that an advance directive is not necessary until one reaches old age. The cases of Quinlan, Cruzan, and Schiavo, however, serve as a compelling counterpoint.

Find and download your state's (if in the U.S.) advance directive form here: https://www.caringinfo.org/planning/advance-directives/by-state/

Multimedia Resources

1 View Brittany Maynard's story as an advocate of the Right to Die movement here: https://www.youtube.com/watch?v=yPfe3rCcUeQ
2 Watch the PBS film *Being Mortal*, featuring Dr. Atul Gawande (referenced in this chapter): https://www.pbs.org/wgbh/frontline/documentary/being-mortal/?utm_source=YouTube&utm_medium=Film&utm_campaign=How_Doctors_Tell_Patients_Theyre_Dying&utm_content=comment/&utm_source=YouTube&utm_medium=Film&utm_campaign=How_Doctors_Tell_Patients_Theyre_Dying&utm_content=comment/

References

American Medical Association. (2026). *Ethics committees in health care institutions* (Opinion 10.7). In *AMA Code of Medical Ethics*. Retrieved January 15, 2026, from https://code-medical-ethics.ama-assn.org/ethics-opinions/ethics-committees-health-care-institutions

Annas, G. J. (1990). Nancy Cruzan and the right to die. *New England Journal of Medicine*, *323*(10), 670–673.

Ariès, P. (1974). *Western attitudes toward death: From the middle ages to the present* (P. M. Ranum, Trans.). Johns Hopkins University Press.

Baile, W. F., Buckman, R., Lenzi, R., Glober, G., Beale, E. A., & Kudelka, A. P. (2000). SPIKES—a six-step protocol for delivering bad news: Application to the patient with cancer. *The Oncologist*, *5*(4), 302–311.

Beauchamp, T. L., & Childress, J. F. (1979). *Principles of biomedical ethics*. Oxford University Press.

Biehl, J. (2005). *Vita: Life in a zone of social abandonment*. University of California Press.

Buchbinder, M., Arora, K. S., McKetchnie, S. M., & Sabbath, E. L. (2024a). Sources of moral distress among obstetrician-gynecologists after Dobbs: A qualitative, multi-state study. *SSM-Qualitative Research in Health*, *6*, 100483.

Buchbinder, M., Browne, A., Berlinger, N., Jenkins, T., & Buchbinder, L. (2024b). Moral stress and moral distress: Confronting challenges in healthcare systems under pressure. *The American Journal of Bioethics*, *24*(12), 8–22.

Coelho, R., Maher, J., Gaind, K. S., & Lemmens, T. (2023). The realities of medical assistance in dying in Canada. *Palliative & Supportive Care*, *21*(5), 871–878.

Frank, A. W. (1995). *The wounded storyteller: Body, illness, and ethics*. University of Chicago Press.

Gawande, A. (2014). *Being mortal: Medicine and what matters in the end.* Metropolitan Books.
Government of Canada. (n.d.). *Canada's medical assistance in dying (MAID) law.* Department of Justice Canada. Retrieved June 29, 2026, from https://www.justice.gc.ca/eng/cj-jp/ad-am/bk-di.html
Grisso, T., & Appelbaum, P. S. (1998). *Assessing competence to consent to treatment: A guide for physicians and other health professionals.* Oxford University Press.
Hamblin, J. (2015, January 25). *The fallacy of "giving up." The Atlantic.* https://www.theatlantic.com/health/archive/2015/01/dying-better/384626
Hannig, A. (2022). 'Assisted suicide' deserves a different name. Here's why. BrandeisNOW. Brandeis University. https://www.brandeis.edu/now/2022/july/assisted-dying-hannig.html
House, S. A., Schoo, C., & Ogilvie, W. A. (2025, May 5). *Advance directives.* In *StatPearls [Internet].* StatPearls Publishing. Retrieved January 6, 2026, from https://www.ncbi.nlm.nih.gov/books/NBK459133/
Jackson Levin, N., Kattari, S. K., Piellusch, E. K., & Watson, E. (2020). "We just take care of each other": Navigating 'chosen family' in the context of health, illness, and the mutual provision of care amongst queer and transgender young adults. *International Journal of Environmental Research and Public Health, 17*(19), 7346.
McGrath, P., Patton, M. A., McGrath, Z., Olgivie, K., Rayner, R., & Holewa, H. (2006). 'It's very difficult to get respite out here at the moment': Australian findings on end-of-life care for Indigenous people. *Health & Social Care in the Community, 14*(2), 147–155.
Middleton, C. (2019). Organ donation after MAiD: It's not that simple. *Canadian Medical Association Journal, 191*(38), E1062.
Snyder, L. (2001). Bioethics, assisted suicide, and the "right to die". *Annals of Clinical Psychiatry, 13*(1), 13–18.
Stonecipher, M. (2006). The evolution of surrogates' right to terminate life-sustaining treatment. *AMA Journal of Ethics, 8*(9), 593–598.
Taub, S. (2001). Commemorative Issue: "Departed, Jan 11, 1983; At Peace, Dec 26, 1990". *AMA Journal of Ethics, 3*(11), 411–413.
ten Have, H., & Patrão Neves, M. D. C. (2021). Right to die. In H. ten Have & M. do C. Patrão Neves (Eds.), *Dictionary of global bioethics* (pp. 929–930). Springer International Publishing.
Weijer, C. (2005). A death in the family: Reflections on the Terri Schiavo case. *CMAJ, 172*(9), 1197–1198.
Weston, K. (1997). *Families we choose: Lesbians, gays, kinship.* Columbia University Press.
Wittenberg, E., Goldsmith, J. V., Buller, H., & Ferrell, B. (2018). Communication in palliative nursing (2nd ed.). Oxford University Press
Yang, C.-H., Wu, C.-Y., Cheng, S.-Y., Mori, M., Suh, S.-Y., Kim, S.-H., Lin, W.-Y., Yamaguchi, T., Huang, H.-L., Hamano, J., Hiratsuka, Y., Tsuneto, S., Morita, T., Chen, P.-J., & the EASED Investigators. (2025). Reasons for and congruence between preferred and actual place of death among cancer patients receiving end-of-life care: A cross-cultural multicenter prospective cohort study in East Asia. *Cancers, 17*(13), 2062.

8 Toward an Integrated, Interdisciplinary, and Collaborative Global Health Communication Paradigm

Introduction

As the very beginning chapter of this book emphasized, the medical humanities and the field of health communication arose out of a distinct need. Scholars, researchers, and activists working within these areas of study were responding to medicine's longstanding history of paternalism and authoritative overreach. Ironically, as we write this present chapter, the authority of medicine, and science and technology at large, is currently being threatened. Unprecedented reports of measles outbreaks across the world have also emerged. In 2024, the U.K. recorded 2,911 measles cases in England, prompting the nation to effectively lose its measles-free status with the WHO (UK Security Agency, 2025). In the U.S., several areas in Texas have so many recorded new measles cases that they are in danger of losing herd immunity (Simpson, 2025). Yet, the resurgence of diseases once believed functionally eradicated does not pertain to the efficacy of the vaccine, but is directly attributable to a rise in the number of parents declining measles, mumps, and rubella (MMR) vaccines for their children. And the driving force behind declining the vaccine is a growing skepticism of medicine.

"Growing" is indeed an accurate way to describe this public movement. Anecdotal reports from obstetricians and pediatricians in our professional circles have indicated that they are witnessing more parents declining a vitamin K injection—to help with clotting until the infant can produce enough of the vitamin on its own—and then electing for a procedure like a circumcision, a combination which places the infant at a much higher risk of a bleeding event. The providers we spoke to speculate that such hesitancy to receive the injection lies in misunderstandings that interpret the injection as another vaccine or also simply not medically necessary and therefore as yet another example of medical overreach. It turns out that these local observations and reports are part of a broader pattern of medical skepticism well-documented in the literature (see Loyal & Shapiro, 2020; Sahni et al., 2014).

Some might say that the public's response represents an inevitability, given medicine's history of paternalism and its historical mistreatment of

DOI: 10.4324/9781003654308-8

certain vulnerable populations, as described in Chapter 1. Surely, there is some validity to this statement, but a view that chalks up medical skepticism to paternalism would be inherently myopic. The public's response to medicine, as exemplified by vaccine hesitancy, is a confluence of multiple systems rooted in politics, media, and the public memory.[1] The problems thus typifying modern medicine are not even medical problems, per se, but as this book has shown, communication problems. In other words, an effective intervention in this regard is not more knowledge, not even more evidence. Instead, it involves recognizing that communication itself transcends multiple systems. Targeting a single system is thus unlikely to effect meaningful change. What the field requires, and what patients deserve, is an approach rooted in a participatory framework, interdisciplinary collaboration, and a **systems-based approach**.[2]

From Paternalistic to Participatory Healthcare

In many ways, a **participatory framework** in medicine runs directly counter to paternalism. As the name suggests, it invites communities and patients to participate in the design and delivery of their own healthcare (Carman et al., 2013). An illustrative example of what a participatory framework might look like in practice is the University of North Carolina-Chapel Hill's (UNC-CH) Formerly Incarcerated Transition (FIT) program (University of North Carolina Department of Family Medicine, n.d.). Eschewing a top-down approach to healthcare, the FIT program is a joint venture among community leaders, healthcare providers, and formerly incarcerated individuals that aims to facilitate societal re-entry for those formerly involved in the carceral or legal systems. But rather than having healthcare personnel dictate what the community needs, the program has created pathways for the community to voice those needs themselves. By making recent incarceration a requisite for hiring and inclusion in this program, the initiative ensures that the patient population it aims to serve is also composed of the individuals who help determine how best to accomplish those goals.

Community-based approaches to healthcare such as this have proven successful, in large part, because they capitalize on the rapport-building function of communication discussed in Chapter 4. As a review, the report function of communication refers to information transmission (i.e., the delivery and receipt of diagnoses, treatment plans), whereas the rapport function encompasses the relational work that allows such information to flow freely and to be meaningfully received. Participatory approaches to healthcare work on the second of these dimensions by treating patients as collaborators—as co-producers of medical knowledge rather than recipients of it. The latter of these functions moreover directly enables the former, leading to improved health outcomes for populations that have historically experienced markedly poorer ones (Wallerstein & Duran, 2010).

The FIT program, and other initiatives like it, capitalizes on the inherent power of the patient-provider concordance discussed in Chapters 2 and 3. The FIT program recognizes that there is reassurance in patients seeing that the individuals steering the course of their healthcare trajectory have been on a similar path at one point in their lives. Admittedly, however, patient-provider concordance is an ideal that is not implementable in every case. It is not feasible for every patient and every provider to share similar life experiences, and this is where the cultural competence discussed in Chapter 2, coupled with reflexive questioning, enters.

Another trend in medicine over the past few decades involves what scholars have dubbed "**medical voluntourism** (Figure 8.1)." Medical voluntourism is where healthcare providers temporarily travel to low- or middle-income countries to provide clinical services in what are often called "mission trips." While often well-intentioned, the brief nature of these trips has led to a broader critique about continuity of care as well, creating sustainable healthcare solutions from within these communities (Maki et al., 2008; Malay, 2017). Medical voluntourism has become so widespread a practice, in fact, that it is an informal requisite of the hidden curriculum (to reference Chapter 5) for applying to medical school. In the U.S. alone, more than 6,000 medical mission trips occur each year, with more than 100,000 healthcare professionals participating (Maki et al., 2008). However, many question the motives behind these initiatives, wondering if they extend beyond seeking an attractive addition to one's curriculum vitae (CV) or professional resume.

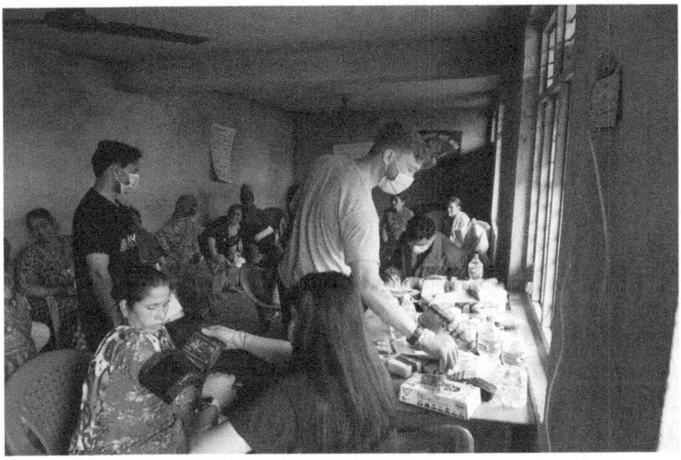

Figure 8.1 A mobile health clinic in Pakistan. Image from Shutterstock.

While the above-described FIT program exemplified the positive effects of communities themselves directing the trajectory of their healthcare, the inverse of this statement may also apply. When those external to certain communities and cultures enter them and then specify the health needs of its members, such an intervention fails more often than not due to the **etic** approach it adopts. An etic approach to understanding a community or culture—their beliefs, customs, daily practices, and even their health needs and goals—adopts an external point of view. It involves the researcher, analyst, or in this case, medical "voluntour" applying their own cultural frame of reference to plan health interventions (Pike, 1967). The mismatch between the community's way of life and the voluntour's is another reason, in addition to the short-term nature of these visits, that leads medical "voluntour" efforts to frequently fail. Chapter 2 of this book, however, emphasizes the importance of an emic approach to providing culturally competent care, whether that be in a local clinic or abroad on a mission trip. In contrast to the etic approach, an **emic** approach to culture and community seeks to understand it from within. Within the context of medical voluntourism, this might look like partnering with community leaders to better understand how existing cultural practices impact health beliefs, as well as how structural constraints influence community members' experiences with illness and disease. Take the example of Guatemala, for instance. Here, many indigenous residents rely on what are termed *comadronas*—traditional birth attendants akin to modern understandings of a doula or non-medical midwife—who provide prenatal and postnatal care, as well as childbirth support. In this cultural context, an emic approach might mean not seeking to replace these traditional birth attendants with Western practitioners, but collaborating with them to learn how pregnancy and childbirth are understood in the community. As this example illustrates, with an emic approach, the goal is not to simply deliver medical services but to embed those services within existing cultural and social structures to meaningfully improve health outcomes.

Healthcare as a Multi-Systemic Undertaking

The social structures alluded to above indeed have a profound effect on both individual and community health. This is why performing a one-time physical exam or administering a single round of vaccinations is unlikely to effect a significant change. Without proper infrastructure in place, this lone physical exam or the course of vaccinations fails to make a dent in addressing health disparities. Acknowledging this fact means also acknowledging that health systems are intricately intertwined with several other systems, economic ones included. In the U.S., where we are writing, health insurance systems are complex. Unlike the single-payer systems in the U.K. and throughout Europe, wherein the national government provides health insurance, most U.S. citizens receive health insurance through their employer. U.S. law stipulates that businesses with more than 500 employees must provide health insurance to their employees. But for those who are self-employed or under-employed (working less than 40 hours a week), accessing health employer-provided health insurance becomes difficult. Additionally, even if one could purchase health insurance through their employer, there is the financial toll of the monthly insurance premium, deductible (the amount the individual must contribute before the insurance company provides reimbursement), and co-pays (the cost-sharing the individual must take on); securing or using health insurance may not be feasible for low-socioeconomic status individuals.

In the U.S., health insurance is a highly politicized issue, which points to how economic and political systems converge to impact citizens' health. Because health spans multiple systems in this way, intervening in one will system will not have a significant impact on health disparities. Therefore, the kind of question practitioners, policymakers, and community health advocates should be asking themselves is how to intervene in a way that touches on multiple systems.

One area of medicine where intersecting systems become especially visible is at the end of life. Decisions regarding hospice referrals, palliative care, and even medically assisted death where permitted are governed not only by the insurance reimbursement schemes outlined above, but by hospital policy, legal frameworks, and longstanding cultural beliefs around quality of life and a "good death." As Chapter 7 of this book articulated, communication is central to navigating these multiple systems. In delivering bad news, for example, clinicians must account for family communication patterns and cultural scripts that may prescribe a more direct or indirect approach. This is where the rapport function of communication described in Chapter 4 enters, however, as clinicians can draw upon the mutual trust they have cultivated through the provider-patient relationship to engage with these moments of profound vulnerability.

Migrant worker health is another example of a multi-systemic issue, spanning politics, economics, and immigration policy. **Migrant workers** are individuals who relocate from one country or region to another for employment (often temporary) to seek greater economic opportunity (International Labour Organization, 2021). The ability of these workers to move across borders, however, is dictated by both economic conditions and immigration policy. The agricultural industry is greatly reliant upon migrant workers, who harvest seasonal produce (Figure 8.2). This type of work is often low-paying and without benefits like health insurance, meaning that it attracts people from other countries where the exchange rate, for example, compensates for a low hourly wage. But immigrating lawfully has proven difficult in political economies throughout the U.S., the U.K., and Europe. In the U.K., for example, prior to Brexit, the U.K. relied heavily on the free flow of European migrant workers. Following Brexit, however, it has had to create the Seasonal Worker Visa to address labor shortages, but this visa offers no long-term pathway to residency or citizenship

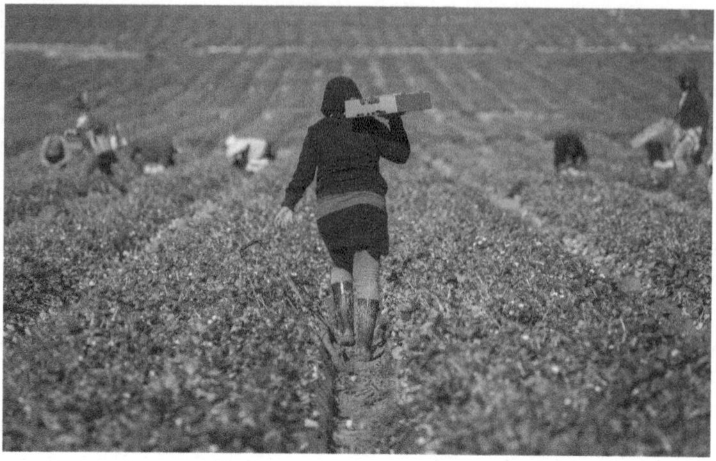

Figure 8.2 Migrant workers picking strawberries in a field. Photo from Shutterstock.

(BBC News, 2018). The EU, too, relies on migrant workers from Eastern Europe and North Africa, many of whom likewise have precarious legal status, unstable housing, and a lack of access to affordable healthcare (Rechel et al., 2011). In the U.S., immigration issues have been at the fore of the public discourse, especially as Immigration and Customs Enforcement (ICE) agents have been dispatched to multiple cities to remove undocumented residents (Griffin & Marcius, 2026). When taken together, these various examples illustrate the fact that migrant worker health—and health in general—cannot be understood as an exclusively medical issue, but as the product of interconnected economic and political systems that influence who is eligible for care.

Migrant worker health is also disproportionately affected by occupational hazards when compared to the rest of the population, which alludes to how **environmental health** and individual health overlap. Environmental health refers to how environmental factors like water supply, air quality, chemical exposures, climate change, and even food supply chains impact human health (WHO, 2023). Referring specifically to chemical exposures, one can see how pesticides that affect environmental health by entering water supplies through agricultural runoff, for example, affect both the public health at a population level and the individual health of migrant workers. In addition to performing repetitive motions that cause musculoskeletal strain (see May et al., 2008), migrant workers are frequently exposed to pesticides and other chemical agents with well-documented adverse health effects. This is why the Environmental Protection Agency (EPA) established the Worker Protection Standard (WPS) (2026) to mandate safety training for pesticide use, the distribution of protective gear and equipment, and access to decontamination supplies like clean water and soap. Yet, most of these constitute harm reduction practices, suggesting that exposure, no matter how protected, will carry some health risks. The example of migrant worker health therefore demonstrates that health disparities are the outcome of multiple interacting systems—environmental, economic, political, and more.

As this discussion suggests, globalization has facilitated border crossing and mobility, but with that has come new healthcare challenges, which invites that perennial question of what providers can do. On a larger scale, many healthcare professionals can and do engage in some form of advocacy work like lobbying, writing scholarly commentaries, and policy advising. But as Chapter 6 notes that the ever-expanding scope of clinicians' duties has been a primary driver of burnout, physicians should therefore not feel compelled to take on such work. That does not mean they must resign themselves to not helping at all, however. Many academic medical centers have created mobile clinics that go directly to farmworkers, thereby eliminating the burden of transportation and of seeking care during normal clinic hours. Examples include the University of North Carolina's Farmworker Health Program (North Carolina Department of Health and Human Services, 2023), Emory University's Farmworker Project (Emory University Rollins School of Public Health, 2023), and the University of Connecticut's Migrant Farmworker Clinic (University of Connecticut School of Medicine, 2023), to name a few. Becoming involved in one of these clinics would represent a way to intervene in the multiple systems impacting human health in a way that does not necessarily lead to burnout.

On an even smaller scale, intervention could mean simply making different language choices in the clinic. As Chapter 3 underscores the notion that language affects perception, and perception, in turn, affects action, being deliberate in the terms one uses to refer to different patient populations can be highly consequential. For example, favoring "undocumented worker" "or out-of-status individual" in lieu of "illegal alien" or even "illegal" signals a certain degree of respect and acknowledgment of humanity that the other terms fail to convey. These choices are small and easy to do, thus creating multiple options for healthcare providers to get involved in a way that is sensitive to the demands placed on their time, energy, and cognitive load.

Collaborative, Interdisciplinary Communication: The Example of Global Health Responses

Returning to the topic of environmental health, in our discussions of AI and digital technologies with our students, they consistently express concerns about the environmental costs of powering these advances. In their discussions, students are careful to acknowledge all of the benefits that AI can bring, such as those outlined in Chapter 6 (e.g., reduced administrative burden), but position these benefits as a tradeoff. AI systems require extensive electricity demands and water for cooling, meaning that as digital infrastructures become more deeply embedded in clinical workflows (Strubell et al., 2019), the environmental hazards of medicine in the contemporary age are no longer limited to pharmaceutical pollution, hospital waste, and the electricity requirements necessary to power diagnostic equipment.

The effects of these actions, however, are not regional or even national. Environmental health is something that affects us all. This is why several nations have historically come together to participate in the Paris Climate Agreement and other international initiatives like the Kyoto Protocol to collectively counter and prevent the effects of climate change. It is notable that nations like the U.S. have recently exited the Paris Climate Agreement, leaving many to worry if global leaders will be able to engage in the interdisciplinary and sustained collaboration necessary to engender meaningful change in this regard.

The good news is that we have evidence that researchers, practitioners, and policymakers across various fields, disciplines, and specialties can work together in the interest of public health. During the COVID-19 pandemic, we saw countries across the world pool and share data related to the disease. Epidemiologists, clinicians, data scientists, and public health officials worked together to sequence the virus' genomes to urgently develop vaccines and track infection patterns so as to inform social distancing protocols. Such collaboration positions the open and free flow of communication across parties as key to addressing the most pressing health crises (Figure 8.3).

In these processes of collaboration, though, several of the same communication challenges presented in Chapter 5 were highlighted. The COVID-19 pandemic may have represented one of the most compelling examples of time-constrained decision-making to date. People were dying and resources were

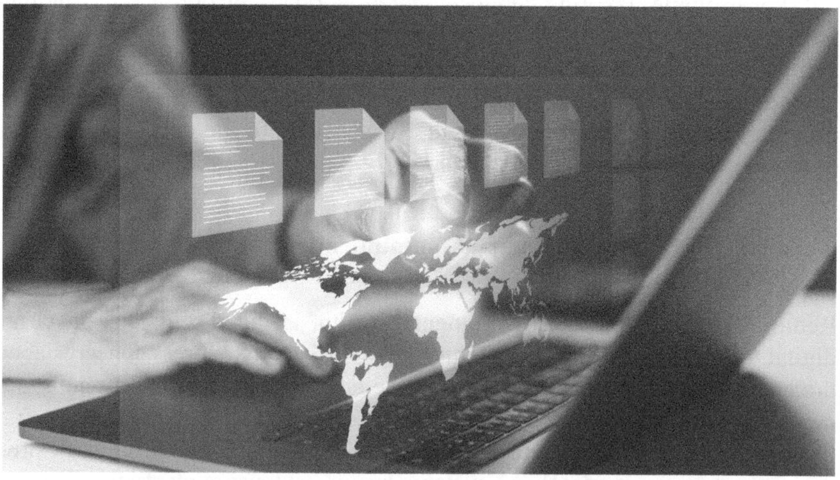

Figure 8.3 A person interacting with global information. Photo from Shutterstock.

limited; clinicians and hospital administrators had to make on-the-fly decisions regarding patient health. The communication in these high-stakes, high-pressure environments shares many of the same qualities as that of individual hospital systems. Just like what is addressed in Chapter 5's discussion of handoffs, where clinicians are tasked with rapidly converting patient stories into actionable knowledge, global responses to the pandemic required public health officials to quickly make sense of evolving scientific evidence so as to deliver it (i.e., to hand it off to) policymakers, healthcare providers, and the public at large. However, Chapter 5 shows this process to be one that is particularly susceptible to communicative breakdowns, and we saw this in the changing masking guidelines, treatment recommendations, and vaccine delivery strategies, all of which was not interpreted by much of the public as difficulty translating information into actionable recommendations, but as evidence of uncertainty and division within the scientific community itself. This perception is, in fact, what gave rise to much of the medical skepticism seen today that was discussed at the beginning of this chapter.

Both organizational hierarchies and the hidden curriculum played out on a global scale during the pandemic as well. Official guidelines regarding lockdown procedures, public health messaging, and vaccine distribution followed a very top-down pathway, as government officials relayed this information to local authorities and then to hospital administrators to ultimately be implemented by frontline healthcare workers. The flow of information in just one direction sedimented many of the hierarchies in place within hospital systems, and moreover prevented a communication learning tool: feedback. Many of the healthcare providers who were closest to patients felt unable—in large part due to the salience and prevalence of these organizational hierarchies—to offer feedback in a way that would inform future policy and action. This example speaks to not just interdisciplinary collaboration but also *lateral* communication—communication that does not move up the chain of command, but instead transcends professional roles, specific institutions, and differing levels of authority. Such communication allows for those closest to patients to share observations and feedback in such a way that public health responses remain grounded in the everyday realities of clinical care.

Finally, the "all hands on deck" mentality that the pandemic cultivated may have worked well to illustrate the power of interdisciplinary and multi-institutional collaboration, but it also revealed the deficits in medicine's hidden curriculum. Professional norms that dictated that healthcare workers persevere amidst pronounced burnout became especially apparent during this time. Healthcare workers felt unprecedented pressure to work under extraordinary conditions, often without sufficient protective gear or resources. However, this expectation was rarely formally communicated through organizational policy, but nonetheless conveyed through a well-established organizational culture of medicine. The key to retaining these professionals, though, is to redefine this organizational culture—to create a culture in which practitioners feel safe to make requests regarding their own safety, to voice concerns, or to simply say "no" to extended working hours.

Medicine's Path Forward

This book has presented cases that illustrate how medicine is practiced within broader, interconnected systems shaped by culture, policy, organizational structures, and perhaps above all, communication dynamics. The cases presented in the book's six analytical chapters show how misunderstandings, mistrust, and even medical mistakes stem not from a lack of scientific knowledge, but in failures in how that knowledge is interpreted, translated, and then implemented. At the same time that communication practices can be a source of these breakdowns, these cases have likewise demonstrated that they can also be the remedy. Clinical communication that attends to the influences of power, culture, and context can provide for not only more effective care, but more equitable care as well.

For the healthcare students, trainees, and practitioners reading this book, the takeaway is quite clear: practicing what Osler (as cited in Rysavy, 2013) identifies as the "art of medicine" (rather than the science of it) requires much more than diagnostic expertise and technical aptitude. It also necessitates that one embrace uncertainty, communicate across disciplinary and cultural boundaries, and remain responsive to the relational and interaction dimensions of care. In this way, the cases herein presented are not meant to offer definitive conclusions to finite problems; rather, they aim to cultivate a certain habit of reflection—an instinct to always question how language, institutional practices and organizational norms, and broader social structures and discourses impact healthcare decision-making, and by extension, patient well-being.

Looking to the future, medicine's path forward will very likely be one accompanied by even more complex challenges. Advances in digital technologies and artificial intelligence, coupled with interconnected globalized healthcare systems, environmental challenges, and wavering public trust in medicine, will continue to carve the road that medicine must follow. So too, however, will the participatory, systems-oriented, and interdisciplinary approaches outlined here. In utilizing and carefully implementing these frameworks, medicine will continue to keep pace with evolving technologies and new health crises. Yet, amidst all this change, one thing will always remain the same: the quality of healthcare will always depend not only on what clinicians know, but also on how they listen, speak, and work together.

Glossary

- **Systems-based approach**
- **Participatory framework**
- **Medical voluntourism**

- **Etic approach**
- **Emic approach**
- **Migrant workers**
- **Environmental health**

Discussion Questions

1 What do you see as the greatest challenge confronting medicine? How do you envision practitioners will solve it?
2 What would a medical "voluntourism" trip need to move from voluntourism to volunteerism? Are there conditions that need to be met to distinguish one from the other?

Further Reading

1 For a precursor to the global cooperation witnessed during the COVID-19 pandemic, read about how public health researchers and medical experts throughout the world worked together to eradicate smallpox in *House on Fire: The Fight to Eradicate Smallpox*: https://www.amazon.com/House-Fire-Eradicate-Smallpox-California/dp/0520274474
2 This article by the BBC's David Grimes positions vaccine skepticism as far from a new phenomenon, but as part of a much older social trend. Read about it here: https://www.bbc.com/future/article/20250905-the-strange-history-of-the-anti-vaccine-movement
3 Read an ethical viewpoint on medical voluntourism featured in the *AMA Journal of Ethics*: https://journalofethics.ama-assn.org/article/voluntourism/2019-09

Multimedia Resources

1 For more information about UNC-CH's FIT program, visit this link: https://www.med.unc.edu/psych/cecmh/services/clinical-services/reach/fit/
2 This video from the Migrant Workers Project provides a summary of many of the barriers to care experienced by this population: https://www.youtube.com/watch?v=eyRi28m0Zos

Exercise

1 You are working as a pediatrician in an outpatient clinic. New parents come in with their infant for the one-month well-child appointment. They are adamantly declining all scheduled vaccinations. Beyond simply educating them on the science of the vaccine itself, and its safety, how else can you navigate this conversation?

Notes

1 The generations that witnessed the toll of diseases like polio that were functionally eradicated by vaccines are now advanced in age. The public memory of the horrors of this disease is thus being forgotten, prompting the public to essentially "forget" the tangible benefits vaccines can bring.

2 A **"systems-based" approach** understands health outcomes as the product of interactions among multiple interconnected elements (e.g., clinical practice, healthcare policy, institutional norms, and communication infrastructure), rather than the result of isolated individual decisions (Leischow et al., 2008; Meadows, 2008).

References

BBC News. (2018, September 6). UK immigration: No visas for low-skilled workers after Brexit. https://www.bbc.com/news/uk-45429397

Carman, K. L., Dardess, P., Maurer, M., Sofaer, S., Adams, K., Bechtel, C., & Sweeney, J. (2013). Patient and family engagement: A framework for understanding the elements and developing interventions and policies. *Health Affairs*, *32*(2), 223–231.

Emory University Rollins School of Public Health. (2023). *Farmworker health research and outreach*. https://www.sph.emory.edu

Griffin, A., & Marcius, C. R. (2026, February 13). *Beyond the big cities, ICE is rattling small-town and exurban America. The New York Times*. https://www.nytimes.com/2026/02/13/us/ice-small-towns.html

International Labour Organization. (2021). ILO global estimates on international migrant workers: Results and methodology. International Labour Office.

Leischow, S. J., Best, A., Trochim, W. M., Clark, P. I., Gallagher, R. S., Marcus, S. E., & Matthews, E. (2008). Systems thinking to improve the public's health. *American Journal of Preventive Medicine*, *35*(2), S196–S203.

Loyal, J., & Shapiro, E. D. (2020). Refusal of intramuscular vitamin K by parents of newborns: A review. *Hospital Pediatrics*, *10*(3), 286–294.

Maki, J., Qualls, M., White, B., Kleefield, S., & Crone, R. (2008). Health impact assessment and short-term medical missions: A methods study to evaluate quality of care. *BMC Health Services Research*, *8*(1), 121.

Malay, P. B. (2017). Short-term medical missions and global health. *The Journal of Foot and Ankle Surgery*, *56*(2), 220–222.

May, J., Hawkes, L., Jones, A., Burdick, P., Ginley, B., Santiago, B., & Rowland, M. (2008). Evaluation of a community-based effort to reduce blueberry harvesting injury. *American Journal of Industrial Medicine*, *51*(4), 307–315.

Meadows, D. (2008). *Thinking in systems*. Chelsea Green Publishing.

North Carolina Department of Health and Human Services. (2023). *North Carolina Farmworker Health Program*. https://ncfhp.ncdhhs.gov/

Pike, K. L. (1967). *Language in relation to a unified theory of the structure of human behavior* (2nd ed.). Mouton.

Rechel, B., Mladovsky, P., Devillé, W., Rijks, B., Petrova-Benedict, R., & McKee, M. (2011). *Migration and health in the European Union*. McGraw-Hill Education (UK).

Rysavy, M. (2013). Evidence-based medicine: A science of uncertainty and an art of probability. *AMA Journal of Ethics*, *15*(1), 4–8.

Sahni, V., Lai, F. Y., & MacDonald, S. E. (2014). Neonatal vitamin K refusal and nonimmunization. *Pediatrics*, *134*(3), 497–503.

Simpson, S. (2025, May 8). *Texas' measles outbreak is nation's largest since 2000*. Texas Tribune. https://www.texastribune.org/2025/05/08/texas-measles-spread-oklahoma-new-mexico/

Strubell, E., Ganesh, A., & McCallum, A. (2019, July). Energy and policy considerations for deep learning in NLP. In *Proceedings of the 57th annual meeting of the Association for Computational Linguistics* (pp. 3645–3650).

U.S. Environmental Protection Agency. (2026). *Worker Protection Standard (WPS) for agricultural pesticides.* https://www.epa.gov/pesticide-worker-safety/agricultural-worker-protection-standard-wps

UK Health Security Agency. (2025, May 23). *What is measles and why is it so important we're all up to date with our MMR vaccine?* https://ukhsa.blog.gov.uk/2026/01/22/what-is-measles-and-why-is-it-so-important-were-up-to-date-with-our-vaccines-to-protect-against-it/

University of Connecticut School of Medicine. (2023). *Migrant Farmworker Clinic.* https://database.outreach.engagement.uconn.edu/program/191

University of North Carolina Department of Family Medicine. (n.d.). North Carolina Formerly Incarcerated Transition (NC FIT) program. University of North Carolina School of Medicine. https://www.med.unc.edu/fammed/service-to-the-community/clinical-care/formerly-incarcerated-transition-program

Wallerstein, N., & Duran, B. (2010). Community-based participatory research contributions to intervention research: The intersection of science and practice to improve health equity. *American Journal of Public Health, 100*(S1), S40–S46.

World Health Organization. (2023). *Environmental health.* https://www.who.int/health-topics/environmental-health

Index

Note: Page references in *italics* refer to figures and with "n" refer to endnotes.

For Product Safety Concerns and Information please contact our EU representative GPSR@taylorandfrancis.com Taylor & Francis Verlag GmbH, Kaufingerstraße 24, 80331 München, Germany